Slimming World's

everyday
Italian

**Over 120 authentic, healthy
and delicious recipes**

EBURY
PRESS

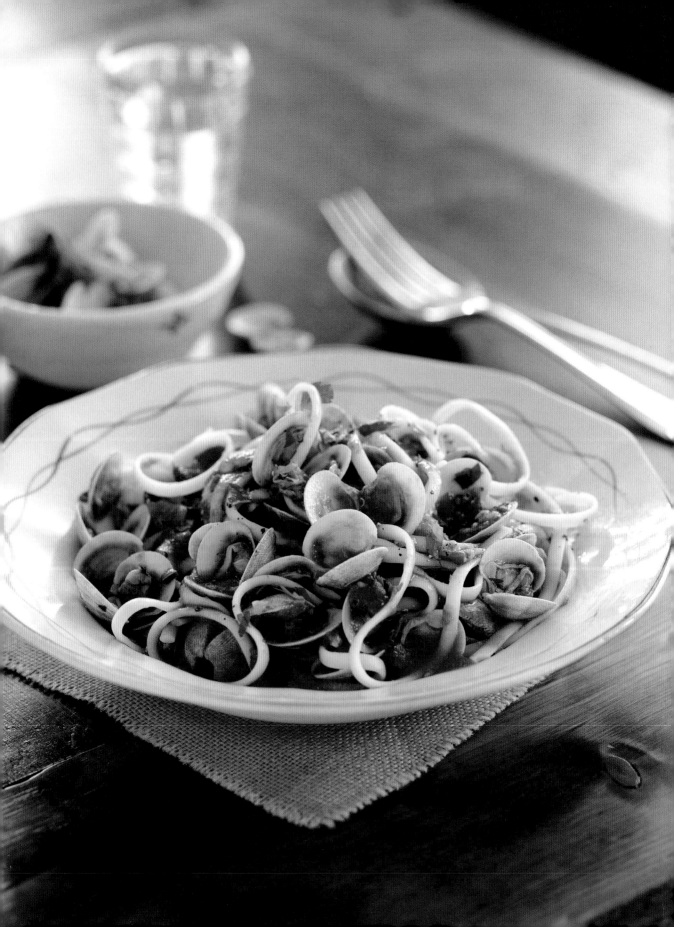

Contents

Cookery notes

Ⓥ Suitable for vegetarians.
❅ Suitable for freezing.

Foreword

Dear reader,
As Slimming World's founder I'm proud to say that we love every opportunity to celebrate. And whenever we get together to share successes and good news, good food is never very far away. So I'm especially pleased to welcome you to *Everyday Italian*, our latest collection of recipes inspired by the food of Italy, where almost every meal is a celebration in itself.

Enjoying food with family and friends is one of life's true pleasures. But for many people struggling with a weight problem – and I speak as someone who has fought this battle myself for many years – it is a pleasure that they believe they can't enjoy. Being overweight can carry with it so many negative feelings: guilt at enjoying food, resentment at not being able to eat as slim people do, despair at 'blowing the diet' again, fear that others are watching you eat and judging you. It's hardly surprising that for many overweight people, sharing a meal isn't a celebration but an ordeal.

That is why, for more than 40 years now, it's been my personal passion and life goal to change the landscape for overweight people, and to empower them to make easy changes that will help them lose weight safely and happily – and to enjoy food, and life, to the full. It starts with Food Optimising, our world-famous way of eating that turns conventional wisdom about 'dieting' on its head. Instead of banning foods, imposing pointless rules and prescribing fixed meals, Food Optimising sets you free to enjoy the foods you love – whether that's a delicious home-made minestrone, a comforting bowl of pasta or a creamy dessert – or all three!

It seems too be good to be true, that you can eat as much as you like of foods you love, and lose weight – but Food Optimising isn't magic; it's based on sound scientific research into how our appetite works and how we can satisfy it without gaining weight. At Slimming World we also have a deep psychological understanding of how it feels to have a weight problem, and how to support and motivate you every step of the way.

Personal, caring support is at the heart of Slimming World's success. Every week in over 6,700 groups in the UK and Ireland, our members find a unique blend of friendship, information and motivation with people who truly understand how they feel, led by a highly trained Consultant who has personal experience of the challenges they face.

In the supportive surroundings of a group, members can celebrate their successes and learn to understand themselves better if things haven't gone so well. If that sounds downbeat and serious, it isn't: there's always plenty of fun and laughter at a Slimming World meeting, and very often the chance to sample favourite recipes and snacks, made by members and brought in to share.

So it's hardly surprising that there is always an air of celebration about a Slimming World group. Week after week, people who thought that they would never be able to lose weight discover that they can – more easily and enjoyably than they ever thought possible. And as they lose weight, they gain confidence and find that they can become the person they always dreamed they could be.

If you're already a member of our Slimming World family, I hope that you will love adding this new collection of fabulous Italian recipes to your Food Optimising repertoire and that it brings you even more joy and success on your journey. If you're new to Slimming World, I hope it will open the door to a whole new approach to weight loss – one that's more liberating, more successful, more fun – than you could ever have dreamed of.

As an old Italian saying has it: 'We are each of us angels with only one wing, and we can only fly by embracing one another.' We look forward to welcoming you to Slimming World soon; let us help you fly!

With warmest wishes

Margaret Miles-Bramwell,
OBE, HonMUniv, FRSA
Founder and Chairman

Introduction

Welcome to *Everyday Italian*, Slimming World's latest collection of mouth-watering recipes that are a delight to cook and to eat, and wonderfully effective at helping you to lose weight and treat the whole family to healthier eating.

Italian cooking ticks every box for food lovers, with its glorious colours, delicious aromas, exciting flavours and – of course – hearty portions. Juicy plum tomatoes, aromatic basil, super fresh seafood and comforting bowls of pasta – it's no wonder we love Italian food. What's more, we associate Italian food with sharing, celebrations, time with friends, family and even romance and glamour. To Italians, food is far more than just fuel; cooking and eating meals together are at the heart of family and social life. It's no wonder that so many of us love to conjure up that spirit of *la dolce vita* (the sweet life) when we buy, cook or eat Italian food.

Italian food is also the perfect choice for a Slimming World recipe collection because we're all food lovers too! Unlike other weight-loss organisations, we've always believed that a love of food and a healthy appetite are to be celebrated and enjoyed, not disciplined and denied. So the Italian style of eating, where food is slowly savoured and enjoyed, is completely in keeping with Food Optimising's approach to eating well to reach and maintain a healthy weight.

That said, much of the Italian-style food we buy in the UK is far from slimmer friendly. Many takeaways and fast foods, in particular, are very different from their Italian originals, and are far less healthy as a result. Pizza, for example, started life in Naples as a thin, crispy snack topped with slivers of cheese, tomato and herbs – a far cry from the monsters laden with high-fat toppings that we see today – and traditional pasta dishes do not swim in oil, cream and cheese.

Because of this, many people still believe that Italian staples, such as pasta and rice, are 'fattening' foods and should be avoided by anyone trying to slim. In fact, cooked with little or no fat, these are filling foods that are relatively low in calories and, as such, they are Free Foods at Slimming World, which means you can eat as much of them as you like – and still lose weight. Thousands of our successful members would agree with the famous Italian beauty Sophia Loren, who has said, 'Everything you see, I owe to spaghetti!'

Back to basics

As we've seen, the secret of eating well and losing weight Italian-style is in the cooking, so in this *Everyday Italian* collection we have gone back to basics. Of course, you'll still find creamy delights such as tiramisu or spaghetti carbonara – using clever lower-fat cooking methods to ensure you can enjoy them without all the calories. But you'll also discover lots of different ways to prepare meals and to flavour them with fresh herbs and seasonings, which are not only healthier, but also bring out the true flavour of the ingredients.

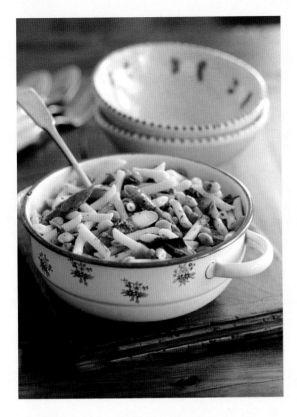

Research is also showing us that we can learn some valuable lessons in health from the traditional Italian way of eating. People who follow a Mediterranean diet, which typically includes plenty of fresh fruit and vegetables, whole grains, lean meat, fish and nuts, with a little olive oil, dairy produce, and even a regular glass of wine, have been found to have a lower risk of developing conditions like heart disease and certain cancers than those who eat a diet with more saturated fat. By cooking the recipes in this book, as part of your Food Optimising plan, you'll naturally be incorporating more of these good habits into your diet.

At a time when many of us are concerned about how to teach our children to enjoy a good relationship with food and to grow up healthy and fit, the Italian tradition of gathering round the table for a leisurely meal is the ideal opportunity for quality family time. Getting the children to help make pizza or meatballs is good fun and will stand them in good stead for later life – and everyone will love the results.

Flavoursome food

If you're an experienced cook, you'll love the opportunity to discover new flavour combinations and Italian regional specialities in this new collection. How about Red Wine Risotto, Balsamic Vinegar Poached Poussins, or Watermelon and Mandarin Granita? And with over 120 delicious dishes to choose from you'll never be bored. But even if you're new to cooking, you'll be surprised at how quick and easy it can be to put together a really impressive meal. Italian cooking at its best is more about marrying ingredients together quite simply, for maximum flavour, rather than complicated cooking techniques.

But the very best thing about *Everyday Italian* is that all the recipes have been designed to fit in beautifully with Slimming World's Food Optimising plan – the world-famous way of eating well to lose weight, feel fantastic and stay slim for life. Turn the page to find out more about how Food Optimising and Slimming World's unique approach to weight management can work for you. And as they say in Italy, *buon appetito*!

For details of a warm and friendly group near you, call 0844 897 8000 or visit www.slimmingworld.com

Food Optimising

Slimming World's Food Optimising plan is a revolutionary and liberating approach to weight loss. It offers a healthy alternative to the traditional approach to 'dieting' based on hunger, deprivation and guilt.

It often seems that most approaches to weight loss treat people either as medical problems that must be fixed, or psychological problems that must be corrected. Slimming World's Food Optimising system is completely different; it starts with a deep understanding of how it feels to be overweight, how daunting it can be to change the habits of a lifetime, and how vital it is to be supported and encouraged during that process.

That's why freedom is at the heart of Food Optimising. All too often, people who want to lose weight feel they are trapped: trapped by feelings of failure each time they fail to stick to a diet, by a fear of going hungry if they cannot satisfy their appetite, and by feeling that they are on a treadmill of dieting, overeating and dieting again that they cannot escape. And the more restrictive a weight loss plan, the more traps lie in wait to make those feelings even worse. It's a vicious circle.

Feel the freedom

So Slimming World introduces members to the idea of enjoying a whole new sense of freedom around food. This includes the promise of never feeling hungry; Food Optimising encourages you to eat to satisfy your appetite, so you never have to worry about when or what your next meal will

be. After years of counting every mouthful, or running out of their food allowance for the day on a set diet, many members find that this freedom is enough on its own to set them on the path to success.

Food Optimising is also about freedom of choice: no foods are banned, there are no set menus and no rules about not eating carbohydrates after lunch or protein if it's Wednesday. There is no need for the iron willpower that so many diet plans require. Instead, Slimming World members learn to give free rein to their choice power – the wonderful freedom to feel confident and in control of healthy eating habits, rather than feeling that food is in control of them.

Naturally, this means making different choices from the ones that have led to having a weight problem. There is no way you can escape from the basic science of the 'energy equation', which is that to lose weight you have to take in fewer calories in food than you expend in activity. But as Slimming World members discover to their delight, that doesn't mean eating less or giving up your favourite foods, or having to eat separate meals from family and friends, and having to turn your life upside down to fit in with some tough new regime.

By sharing tips and ideas in their group, finding out about healthier ways to shop

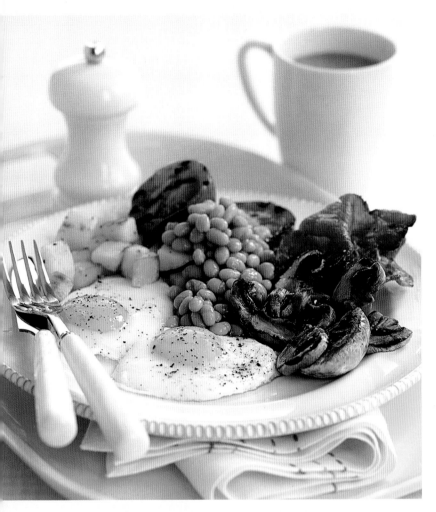

many members tell us that Food Optimising is cheaper than the way they ate before). Instead, at Slimming World, a 'Free' food or recipe is simply one that you can eat freely – as much as you like to satisfy your appetite, whenever you like. There is no counting, no measuring, just delicious food to enjoy without feeling guilty or worrying about overeating.

There are hundreds of Free Foods to choose from when you're Food Optimising, and they include those foods that we all eat every day – fruit and vegetables, lean meat, fish and poultry, eggs, pulses and fat free dairy produce. Free Foods are those that have been found to satisfy our appetite without being packed with fat and calories. So by filling up on Free Foods every day (and Superfree Foods, which are even more slimmer-friendly), you naturally reduce your energy intake without going hungry or having to count every bite. For more about Free and Superfree Foods, see pages 12–13.

Free Foods are the cornerstone of Food Optimising's success as an effective and enjoyable way of managing your weight. It isn't a diet (remember, DIET stands for Dare I Eat That?), but a healthy lifestyle.

It was easy to create a whole book of Italian recipes, Slimming World style, because so many of everyone's favourite Italian foods are Free when you're Food Optimising. Stock up on dried pasta, rice, beans and pulses, for example: all these

and cook and learning how to cope with the challenges they face in using their choice power to best effect, members overwhelmingly find that the only changes they experience are positive ones – having more energy, enjoying food even more, and achieving the weight and shape they want to be.

And they achieve all this by Food Optimising, following an easy three-step series of choices: Free Foods, Healthy Extras and Syns.

Fabulous Free Foods

If you're new to Slimming World and look at the recipes in *Everyday Italian*, you'll see that many of them are 'Free'. This doesn't mean that they cost nothing (although

Italian staples are Free and help make filling, delicious meals. Fresh and frozen fish and seafood, which feature in so many Italian classics, are Free too, and so are all kinds of lean meat and poultry, so you can ring the changes with beef, veal, chicken, pork, ham and game whenever you like. Whip up a tasty frittata (Italian omelette) with plenty of eggs – they're Free too – and, of course, pile on the vegetables, fruit and fat free dairy produce. All the ingredients you need for a rich tomato sauce, a peperonata (warm pepper salad) or a minestrone soup – and hundreds of other Italian delights besides – are Free Foods at Slimming World.

Healthy Extras
And there is even more to Food Optimising than Free Foods! Slimming World members quickly discover that they have even more choices in the form of Healthy Extras and Syns – two important components that ensure that Food Optimising is the healthiest, most generous and most flexible system you will find.

Each day, in addition to all those Free Foods, you can choose from a long list of Healthy Extras – foods that are either high in fibre or rich in essential nutrients, such as calcium. Wholemeal bread, soup, dried or tinned fruit, milk and cheese, breakfast cereal and cereal bars, olive oil, and more besides, are all on the Healthy Extras list that Food Optimisers can enjoy at any time through the day. For more about Healthy Extras, see page 14.

The joy of synergy
And then last, but just as important in their own way, are Syns. The word Syns comes from 'synergy', which describes what happens when things work so much better together than they would on their own. Every day, on top of Free Foods and Healthy Extras, Food Optimisers can choose between 5 and 15 Syns to use whenever and however they like. Foods that have a high Syn value tend to be those that we don't need much of, such as fatty, sugary and processed foods, and alcohol. You can Food Optimise and lose weight easily without using Syns at all, but many, many members find that they are key to their long-term success. Knowing that you can enjoy chocolate every day, or cream on your fruit salad, or a packet of crisps, without feeling guilty, can make all the difference between feeling that you are 'on a diet' and enjoying a way of eating you can follow for life. For more on Syns see page 15.

Extra Easy, extra choice
Building your daily and weekly menu plans using Free Foods, Healthy Extras and Syns couldn't be easier. Just to make the point, the name for our most popular way of Food Optimising is Extra Easy. It's Food Optimising for the 21st century – offering Slimming World members more freedom and choices than ever.

Extra Easy encourages you to satisfy your appetite each day with a fabulous choice of Free Foods and Superfree Foods, including lean meat and poultry, fish, vegetarian meat alternatives, eggs, all vegetables, pulses, rice, pasta and grains, fresh and frozen fruit, fat free dairy produce, lots of different seasonings and low-calorie drinks. So if you want a huge grilled steak and a big, fluffy jacket potato, go right ahead! A full English breakfast with grilled bacon, scrambled eggs, tomatoes, baked beans and mushrooms? Be our guest! Or a spicy lamb rogan josh with lentil dhal and a pile of boiled rice? Help yourself – and go back for seconds if you like. For fabulous weight loss, we suggest you fill one-third of your plate with Superfree Food for main meals.

As well as all that Free Food, we ask you to make two Healthy Extra choices each day – one that's high in fibre, and one rich in calcium. Here again there are plenty of generous choices, including breakfast cereals and cereal bars, bread and crispbreads, as well as cheese and milk (including non-dairy milk).

And if you can still squeeze in even more, you can choose between 5 and 15 Syns each day, depending on how many you feel would be most helpful to you in reaching your goal.

There are so many reasons why Extra Easy is such a fantastic way to start your journey to success with Slimming World. As you can see, there is literally no limit to the number of meals you can create, so you'll never be bored. It's based on fresh, unprocessed, natural foods that encourage you to cook more, so that you'll know exactly what's going into your meals, and it's cheaper than relying on ready meals and takeaways too. Furthermore, there is so little counting, weighing and measuring to do, that you can forget you're trying to slim from one week to the next – until you step on the scales at your Slimming World meeting and get a very nice surprise!

Building your menus using Free Foods, Healthy Extras and Syns is so, so easy

The Original and Green choices

Extra Easy is a clever mix of Slimming World's two classic 'choices' or styles of menu, the Original choice and the Green choice. Both choices are safe, effective and delicious to follow: it's just a question of basing your meals on the kinds of foods you prefer and that fit your lifestyle best.

The Original choice is for you if you particularly enjoy satisfying, protein-rich foods such as lean meat, poultry, fish, seafood and eggs; on Original you create your meals using these foods, along with all fresh fruit and nearly all vegetables, plus some dairy products such as fat free natural yogurt or fromage frais. Add delicious daily Healthy Extras, such as wholemeal bread and pasta, potatoes, high-fibre breakfast cereals and cheese or milk, then decide how to use your Syns for the day.

And if your favourite foods are the comforting, carbohydrate-rich staples such as pasta, potatoes, rice and pulses – then go Green. Pile your plate with these foods, as well as your pick of fresh fruit and vegetables, eggs and dairy products, such as fat free natural yogurt or fromage frais. Add lean meat or fish as Healthy Extras, if you like, or opt for some wholemeal bread, high-fibre breakfast cereals and cheese or milk, then choose your Syns for the day.

This book can only give you a brief introduction into the wonders of Food Optimising. Once you join a Slimming World group, you'll be amazed at how much more you'll discover.

Free Foods

The idea that you could eat as much as you like of everyday foods and still lose weight was revolutionary over 40 years ago when Slimming World first introduced it to amazed and delighted slimmers. Even now, when nutrition scientists know much more about how our appetite works, many weight loss plans still focus on restriction – small portion sizes, banned foods, strict rules on how foods can be combined, or when you can eat.

Many of these systems use complex scientific terms and claims as if to convince us that the more complicated a diet is, the more effective it will be. Food Optimising is the opposite – it is beautifully simple and yet the science it is based on is completely sound.

Feel fuller for longer

At Slimming World, Free Foods are those that have been found by research to keep us feeling fuller for longer. Of the major food groups, we know that foods high in protein, such as lean meat, fish and eggs, or foods rich in carbohydrates, like pasta, potatoes and rice, are most effective in satisfying our appetite. This is because they either trigger the signal that stops us eating when the body doesn't need any more (satiation) or the signal that prevents us from wanting to eat again until we need more energy (satiety).

Foods from the other food groups, such as fat, and alcohol, are far less effective in satisfying appetite. Many foods that are rich in carbohydrates or protein are extra-effective for slimmers because they are low in energy density, which means that weight for weight, they are relatively low in calories. For example, a large jacket potato may weigh many times more than a small bar of chocolate, but may have the same number of calories. Low energy dense foods also tend to be bulky, which makes it harder to overeat on them, while high energy-dense foods – such as those that have a lot of fat or oil, or are highly processed – are much quicker and easier to eat without triggering all the signals that truly satisfy your appetite.

There are many reasons why basing your meals on Free Foods is so powerful and effective in helping you lose weight:

- You'll be automatically limiting your calorie intake, without counting a single calorie.
- You'll feel less need for high-sugar, high-fat snacks that pile on calories without providing much nutritional benefit.
- Most Free Foods are natural, unprocessed foods without lots of added ingredients, so you can create your own healthy meals and know exactly what you and your family are eating.
- Free Foods are delicious!

Superfree, super filling foods

Some foods that are extra-helpful to slimmers, because they are especially low in energy density, are called Superfree at Slimming World. Filling a third of your plate with Superfree Foods at every meal can give your weight loss a welcome boost when you're following the Extra Easy plan. And we're not talking lettuce leaves and grapefruit. Superfree Foods include fresh and frozen fruit and most vegetables and make boosting your weight loss a pleasure not a chore.

Free Foods are the key that helps Slimming World members switch on their 'choice power' and set themselves free from the tyranny of feeling hungry, bored or self-conscious about what they're eating while they are on their weight-loss journey. And because Free Foods are the basis of the healthy diet that's recommended for everyone, Free Foods are also the passport to a lifetime of delicious eating, Slimming World style.

Your Free Foods questions answered

Q I don't like fruit or vegetables. Can I still Food Optimise properly?

A Yes, of course. There are so many Free Foods on the list that you're bound to find some to satisfy your appetite, whatever your likes and dislikes. That said, we all know that eating fruit and vegetables is important for health, and they will fill you up too, so they're hugely valuable to slimmers. Slimming World has hundreds of ideas to make fruit and vegetables tasty and exciting – you might surprise yourself.

Q Why aren't fruit juice and smoothies Free Foods, if they only contain fruit?

A Most Free Foods take time to chew and eat, activating all the signals the body sends to the brain to indicate that it is full. Think how quickly you can drink a glass of apple juice compared with eating two or three whole apples; the much more energy-dense juice is gone before you know it, and you won't have benefited from the soluble fibre in the apple flesh and skin. Smoothies do include fruit flesh, but because they contain a lot of calories for their volume, they do not count as Free.

Q Can I overeat on Free and Superfree Foods?

A No, definitely not! It's important to be confident that you can satisfy your appetite without worrying about going hungry. Many people new to Food Optimising find it hard to believe that they can eat as many Free Foods as they like, and test it to the limit. They find it even more amazing the next week when they find they have lost weight while piling their plate high at each meal.

Healthy Extras

As their name suggests, Healthy Extras are Slimming World's way of ensuring that you have a little extra help in achieving a way of eating that's healthy as well as effective for weight loss.

Each day, in addition to unlimited Free Food, we ask you to make choices from a list of Healthy Extras: with the Extra Easy plan, it's two choices each day. You're asked to measure your Healthy Extras, because they aren't as low in energy density as Free Foods, but they are extra-useful for slimmers in other ways.

For example, Healthy Extra 'a' choice foods are rich in vitamins and minerals, especially calcium, which is vital for strong bones and teeth, and it also helps nerves, muscles and blood to function properly, protects against high blood pressure and may even play a role in helping the body metabolise body fat. Many Free Foods contain calcium, and having calcium-rich milk (including dairy-free alternatives) or cheese every day as a Healthy Extra choice is an easy way of helping your intake.

Healthy Extra 'b' choices are designed to increase the amount of fibre we eat. Eating plenty of fibre is important for health, as it helps keep our digestive system working efficiently. The soluble fibre found in fruit and oats can also help to lower cholesterol and so reduce our risk of heart disease. Fibre-rich foods are slimmer friendly because they are often bulky, which means they're a good way of filling up. Many Free Foods, such as fruit and vegetables, contain fibre, but many of us enjoy high-fibre breakfast cereals, wholemeal bread

or beans and pulses as our major fibre providers. Having a Healthy Extra 'b' choice each day ensures you can eat in the way that suits you – for example, a bowl of bran cereal for breakfast, a sandwich for lunch or a cereal bar as a snack – and still lose weight safely and steadily.

You can enjoy Healthy Extras with meals, as snacks or through the day, for example by having milk in cups of tea or coffee.

Your Healthy Extras questions answered

Q What if I don't have time to weigh and measure my Healthy Extras?

A No problem! You'll find 'Grab & Go' choices on the list for when you have time to eat, but not to weigh. These include pre-packed cheese portions, crispbreads, cereals and cereal bars.

Q Do I have to have particular brands of Healthy Extra foods?

A Not if you don't want to. Many Healthy Extras are non-branded foods, so you can use a supermarket own-brand.

Q Do I have to have my Healthy Extras?

A We recommend that you do, to fill you up and for optimum health.

Syns

Syns, the third important element of Food Optimising, are the way that Food Optimising gives you a flexible safety net, so that you can enjoy all the freedom that you need to succeed, with just enough control to safeguard your weight loss each week.

Starting on a weight-loss plan can feel like walking a tightrope: wobble for just a second away from the straight and narrow and you find you've fallen off, with the prospect of a tough climb back to the start again. The more restrictive the plan, the more likely you are to fall into this cycle of failing, blaming yourself and trying again, each time with a little less motivation and self-esteem than before. Free Foods help to spring you out of that trap once and for all and Syns are another part of the plan designed to help you stay on track.

All foods that are not Free have a Syn value; a small packet of crisps or a small glass of wine, for instance, each counts as around 5 Syns. Foods that are high in Syns tend to be the high-fat, high-sugar, highly processed foods that we are all advised to eat less of, and that are most unhelpful if you're trying to lose weight. But, human nature being what it is, these are often the very foods that we are most fond of and would hate to give up completely.

So at Slimming World, you don't have to. Every day, as well as all your Free Food and Healthy Extras, you have 5–15 Syns to use, however you like. The choice is up to you, because everyone is different. Some people, for instance, aren't keen on chocolate but love to nibble on cheese; others don't drink alcohol but think a cup of tea is too wet without a biscuit. You can use your Syns with meals, or at any time as a snack, or when eating out; you might even find you don't have room to use all your Syns every day, and that's fine too.

Your Syns questions answered

Q Can I do without Syns at all?

A From a nutritional point of view, Syns aren't essential, so yes, you can do without them; it's absolutely your choice. But many Food Optimisers find that giving themselves 'permission' to enjoy their Syns is a vital part of breaking out of the diet trap and being able to eat healthily for life, so why deprive yourself?

Q What happens if I have too many Syns?

A Nothing! We all have days when life gets in the way of our good intentions; the secret of success is to put them behind us and start again. There's no need to beat yourself up or try to over-compensate. In your Slimming World group, your Consultant and fellow members will show you how to cope if you have a special occasion coming up when you might like to have more Syns than usual.

15

Image Therapy

At Slimming World we talk a lot about 'synergy' – the magical process by which, when you mix different elements together, they produce results that are much more powerful than they would be on their own. Synergy is a brilliant way to describe what happens in a Slimming World group too, when members and their Consultant get together to achieve goals that they would never have thought possible before they joined.

At Slimming World, the individual member is at the heart of the process. Although you are part of a group, we also promise to listen to and respect you as an individual, recognising that everyone is different and will find their own path to success. It starts when you first walk through our doors; we understand just how hard it can be to take that step, and so before you even take part in the meeting, your Consultant will spend time with you and other new members, talking you through Food Optimising and assuring you of the support and care you can look forward to.

Choose your own target

The individual approach continues as you weigh in for the first time and think about the target you'd like to achieve – and you might be surprised to know that this is entirely up to you. Some new members know exactly what weight they would like to be, others prefer to set an interim goal that's within reach, and some people just want to take it one week at a time. Some people choose a dress size or a waist size they'd like to reach. The important thing is to take the approach that works for you – at Slimming World, you are always in control and take all the big decisions.

What happens in group

All our Consultants are highly trained and have personal experience of battling a weight problem, so you can be absolutely sure that no one will judge you, humiliate you or make embarrassing revelations about your weight. Your weigh-in is private, and your weight is never read out to the group – only the progress you make week by week. In the meeting, everyone in the group receives their share of individual attention, praise and support from their Consultant and fellow members, and has the chance to review how their week has gone and to set a goal for the week to come. Even if you feel you haven't done particularly well, the warmth, friendship and practical tips from the group are a fabulous boost for the next week. And if you are celebrating a success, the applause and congratulations will send you out floating on air.

Being part of a lively, buzzy group of people who all share the same aim, while at the same time benefiting from individual praise, support and help, is amazingly

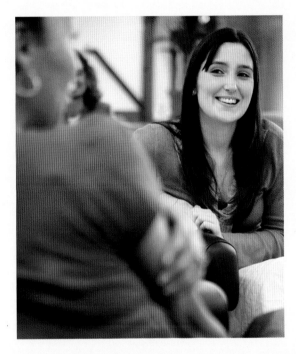

and motivation, which help members identify their own more deep-seated issues around food. This includes helping people to identify patterns of behaviour that may be sabotaging their own success, and working out ways to change those patterns over time.

Image Therapy is also tremendous fun! There's always plenty of laughter in a Slimming World group, and very often there is something exciting going on like a food tasting, a quiz or a chance to enter one of our Slimming World competitions.

And the friendship, resources and support continue between meetings too. Slimming World's website has exclusive content for members, including interactive food diaries, a personalised progress chart and a searchable recipe archive, so you're never short of ideas or inspiration. You can also choose to link up with Lifelines – group members who text, phone or email each other for an extra boost of motivation or to share news.

powerful for our members. We call this Image Therapy, which stands for Individual Motivation And Group Experience. Based on a deep understanding of the psychology of overweight people, this unique support system is designed to increase the confidence and self-esteem of our members, while also equipping them with tools to develop lasting lifestyle changes.

Image Therapy is tailored to meet the needs of individual slimmers, based on the understanding that every overweight person is different, and shaped by a complex mixture of factors. It works on several levels: from offering practical advice and tips, including recipe ideas and ways to avoid common pitfalls, to much deeper levels of support

Synergy is a brilliant way to describe what happens at a Slimming World group

Celebrating along the way

There's nothing like reaching a target to send your motivation soaring, and one goal that Slimming World encourages every member to set is their 'Club 10' target.

You join 'Club 10' when you've lost 10 per cent of your starting weight and have kept it off (or gone on to lose more) for 10 weeks. It's a milestone worth celebrating, because research shows that if you're overweight, losing just 10 per cent of your weight and maintaining it is enough to start seeing important health benefits. It's tremendously motivating to know that, even if you still have a way to go, you've already helped to lower your blood pressure, reduce your risk of developing type 2 diabetes, ease pressure on your joints and lungs, and lower your blood cholesterol – just by losing a modest amount of weight and keeping it off. Members who reach their Club 10 target are rewarded with a free week's membership – and huge respect and applause from everyone in the group.

Reaching your target

Everyone who's tried to lose weight will know that reaching your target weight is just the beginning, but maintaining it is a huge challenge too. Slimming World understands this completely, and knows just how important it is to have support and motivation as you start your new slim life. For this reason, everyone who reaches their target weight – the target you have chosen – is rewarded for their fantastic achievement with free membership for life, just as long as they stay within a few pounds either side of their target. Every group cherishes its target members who go along as often as they like to meet old friends and make new ones. They're a hugely important part of Slimming World, as they are so inspiring to members. So much for the critics who say that the 'diet industry' doesn't want people to succeed!

In fact, a sense of responsibility for the whole family's health and wellbeing has

always been close to Slimming World's heart. Our research has shown that our members, 95 per cent of whom are women, have an important influence on how others in their family circle eat, as the cooking and food shopping very often falls to them. And the great news is that if the primary shopper joins Slimming World, the whole family's diet benefits – 85 per cent of members report buying more fruit and vegetables for the family than before, and 80 per cent say they and their families eat less fatty food than before.

Free2Go

Recently, Slimming World has taken this whole-family approach onto another, even more effective level, by reaching out directly to young people from 11 to 15, who can attend Slimming World free of charge, with the consent of their GP, as long as they are accompanied by a parent or guardian who is willing to help the young person change their lifestyle with the support of the family.

An eating plan designed especially for young people with busy lives, called Free2Go, encourages them to fill up on satisfying food with no counting and measuring. It also takes full account of a teenager's need to have fun with friends, to eat out and, above all, not to feel different from their peers. In the group, the focus is not on the young person's weight but on the positive changes they might have made during the week, with plenty of praise and support for every step in the

> By losing a modest amount of weight and keeping it off, you help to lower your blood pressure and cholesterol and ease pressure on your joints

right direction. The scheme has proved to be a big success and a terrific support to thousands of concerned parents who felt they had nowhere to turn in helping their children to avoid a lifetime of obesity.

Mums-to-be and Food Optimising

As we learn more about the impact of obesity on our health, research places increasing emphasis on the importance of managing weight gain in pregnancy. These days we know that 'eating for two' is not necessary, and that a big weight gain can lead to problems such as gestational diabetes, high blood pressure or a more difficult birth.

It can be very difficult for mums-to-be to keep an eye on their weight while ensuring that they are eating healthily for themselves and their baby, so Slimming World is very proud that we're the only slimming club to offer support to pregnant women. Any woman who wishes to attend Slimming World during her pregnancy needs the consent of her midwife, who will make any recommendations on managing her weight safely. Our policy has been developed with the Royal College of Midwives, and as Food Optimising is based on the same healthy, balanced diet that's recommended for all pregnant women, it is our privilege to help to look after members at this special time in their lives.

Slimming World and the NHS working together

It's not surprising that Slimming World's unique and unbeatable approach to weight management is proving popular with healthcare professionals who are looking for the best ways to help overweight

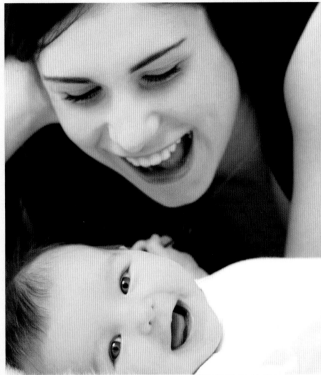

people in their care. Slimming World was the first organisation to offer a 'referral service' to the National Health Service. We are currently working with over 70 NHS Trusts, having shown them the evidence that losing weight with Slimming World is as safe and effective as other methods, such as diet pills or surgery – at a fraction of the cost.

And members who are referred to us via a local Slimming World on Referral scheme pay nothing at all; they are offered 12 weeks' free membership of a local group, after which their GP may refer them for a further 12 weeks or they choose to carry on paying for their own membership. The results have been extremely positive; many members do continue as paying members after their initial experience, and go on to enjoy fantastic success.

Your Image Therapy questions answered

Over 40 years of experience have taught us that no matter where you start on your weight loss journey, and whatever your lifestyle or stage of life, there is no problem that can't be overcome with the help of Slimming World. A uniquely flexible eating plan, a wonderfully effective way of empowering people to make healthy choices, and an exhilarating blend of fun, support and friendship – as our 300,000 members find every week – it's an unbeatable combination. Here are some of your most frequently asked questions.

Q I'm not sure I'll have time to stay to group after being weighed every week. Do I have to?

A No, you don't have to, but if you don't, it's a real shame. You risk missing out on the most valuable part of Slimming World's service to you: the support, enthusiasm, ideas and good fun that are at the heart of every group. Our surveys show that members who take part in Image Therapy as often as they can are more successful than those who don't. So we really do encourage you to stay and make the most of your Slimming World group. It's an hour or so a week that could change your life.

Q If I've had a bad week, isn't it better to stay away and try to sort it out myself?

A It might sound like a good idea, but all our experience tells us that staying away from your group is just storing up more problems for the future. Although it might seem hard to do, you'll feel much better about yourself if you go to your group, think about what might have gone wrong, then draw a line under your bad week and set a fresh goal. Your Consultant and fellow members will be proud of you for turning up – and even prouder when you reach your next milestone. And if you've drifted away from the group and are worried about returning – don't be! Your welcome will be just as warm and the support just as strong.

Q My GP has referred me to my local Slimming World group, but I'm embarrassed in case I'm made to feel different. How will I be treated?

A It's very important that every Slimming World member is made to feel valued and welcome – because you are. No one will be able to tell that you have joined Slimming World via your healthcare professional and if you do choose to share that information with the group, it's entirely up to you.

Q Walking into a room full of strangers is something I normally try to avoid. Will everyone turn and stare?

A Many of our new members are nervous and self-conscious; it's completely understandable. Your Consultant and her team will be looking out for new arrivals and will make sure you're welcomed right away, and there's lots going on at the start of the meeting, so before you know it, you'll feel like part of the crowd.

Body Magic

The more scientists discover about exercise, the more the evidence stacks up that being active really can have an almost magical effect on our health and wellbeing.

Regular moderate activity – at a level that speeds up your heart rate and breathing, but that isn't exhausting – has been shown to have a protective effect against all kinds of serious conditions such as high blood pressure, stroke, heart disease, certain cancers, brittle bones and type 2 diabetes.

More recently, attention has focused on exercise's ability to boost our mood and improve wellbeing. We've probably all heard of endorphins, the feel-good hormones that are released when we exercise. Experts now believe that a 'prescription' of regular exercise can be very helpful for people affected by depression, anxiety and stress.

You might think that you need to be running marathons or playing competitive sport to reap these benefits, but that's not the case. The recommended level of activity to achieve good health is 30 minutes of brisk walking, five days a week. And you don't need to have started young, either: one study found that a group of men who started exercising aged 50 improved their health prospects as much as if they had given up smoking, and similar results have been seen in post-menopausal women.

Exercise is great energy-booster too; it's the gift to yourself that keeps giving back. If you're tired and you don't feel like going for a brisk walk or for a swim, it's hard to believe that exercising will make you feel better. But more often than not, once you get going, you find your energy level rises, and by the time you've finished, you feel refreshed and alert again.

And of course, exercising burns calories, so it is an important part of the 'energy equation', helping you to increase your energy expenditure while at the same time decreasing your energy intake if you're trying to lose weight. When it comes to weight loss, exercise on its own is definitely not a magic bullet; our bodies have evolved to be extremely quick to store energy and extremely slow to spend it, so many of us overestimate the amount of calories we expend in exercise. Even so, adding three to four moderate exercise sessions a week to a healthy eating plan will help you lose around 1–2lb a month more than you would by dieting alone.

So together with a healthy eating plan, exercise is a fantastic way to improve your health, boost your self-esteem and keep your motivation high – all of which will speed your weight loss along.

> Taking regular exercise boosts our mood and improves our sense of wellbeing

Body Magic and you

Despite all the evidence of how valuable exercise is, many of us are not as active as we could be. In fact, a recent Government survey suggests that seven out of 10 women do less than the recommended 30 minutes of activity five times a week. It's clear that knowing that exercise is good for us isn't necessarily enough to make us do it – just as knowing about healthy eating doesn't always mean that we eat well all the time.

So just as Slimming World's approach to food starts with understanding how slimmers feel, our approach to exercise is exactly the same. We call it Body Magic, and it's a way of harnessing the benefits of exercise, together with Food Optimising, for a combined effect that produces magical results.

Just as Food Optimising is about making small changes that lead to permanent changes in eating habits, so Body Magic is about starting from wherever you may be on the 'pathway to activity' and building up steadily so that exercising becomes a part of daily life, as regular as brushing your teeth. We know that some of our members are already keen exercisers when they join us; others may have lost the activity habit years ago or they may have problems that prevent them being very mobile. So a one-size-fits-all exercise programme is not for us.

As with Food Optimising, Body Magic invites members to set their own goals, and choose how they want to reach them, while being supported every step of the way. Each week, members are encouraged to set Body Magic goals that they note down in a private FIT Log (it stands for Frequency, Intensity and Time). This might be for instance, 'walk 30 minutes a day' or 'do my aerobics DVD for two hours this week'.

Reap the rewards

As they gradually build up the amount of time they spend on exercise, members can work towards Body Magic awards, which are earned at different stages:

- Bronze, when you're active for at least 45 minutes each week, spread over at least three days and maintained for four weeks or more.
- Silver, which you reach four weeks after building up to six 15-minute sessions of activity each week, spread over three to five days and maintained for four weeks.
- Gold, achieved when you are being active for ten 15-minute sessions a week, spread over three to five days and maintained for eight weeks. This is the level the Government recommends for maintaining good health.
- Platinum, when exercise and activity are automatic and regular in your weekly routine and you can't imagine life without them.

There is no set time limit for building up through these stages; Body Magic is not just a box-ticking exercise to earn a certificate at the end (although it's a great feeling when you do!). The aim is to help you develop real, life-changing habits that you want to continue forever, and inevitably people will get there at their own speed.

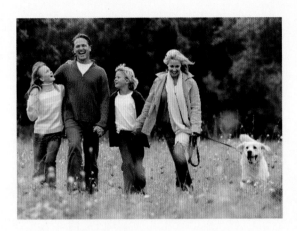

Every little thing you do is magic

We also understand that motivating yourself to exercise can be very challenging; many of us with busy lives have difficulties in finding the time for a gym session, for example, and even if we have time, we may feel self-conscious or nervous about doing formal exercise. All the evidence shows that successful exercisers are those who find something they enjoy and that they can stick to over time, building up that valuable activity habit. Non-formal exercise such as putting extra effort into housework, cleaning the car, gardening or walking the dog can be just as effective as a gym workout or dance class – they all contribute to Body Magic. You don't even need to exercise for 30 minutes at a time – two 15-minute sessions are just as good if time is tight.

In their Slimming World group, members share lots of tips like this on how they find time to exercise – whether it's taking a brisk walk round the block at lunchtime, choosing to go for a swim with a friend instead of to the pictures, or challenging the family to a vigorous fitness video game instead of watching TV.

Your Body Magic questions answered

Q Won't exercising make me feel hungry?

A You might think this would be the case, but in fact, you're less likely to want to eat after you've exercised. And if you do feel peckish after a swim or a gym session, there's no problem when you're Food Optimising: you can satisfy your appetite with Free Foods whenever you like, without undoing all your hard work.

Q I haven't done any sport since schooldays – and I hated it then! What kind of Body Magic is best for me?

A If you don't enjoy playing sports or formal exercise like the gym or an exercise class, you can still improve your fitness and energy with Body Magic. It's about building extra activity into your day: put a bit more effort into the housework, go for a few minutes' walk round the block, dance to a record while cooking the dinner – it will all be beneficial.

Q I'd like to exercise but I can never seem to find the time. What can I do?

A Although you feel you'd like to exercise, it may be quite low on your list of priorities and, if so, there will always be something more urgent to do. Try thinking of exercise time as an important appointment you make with yourself; write it in your diary and don't let anything get in the way. Talk it over with your Slimming World group; they are bound to have some good ideas and tips for squeezing activity into a busy day.

Chapter 1

Soups and starters

Italian meals often start with antipasti, a selection of small dishes that are easily put together and served hot or cold. Our Seafood Antipasto is a classic example (see page 42), but you could mix and match many of our fresh, tasty ideas to make perfect party food as well as stylish first courses.

For colder days we've also included some comforting soups, such as the familiar minestrone with pasta and vegetables, and the more unusual Zuppa alla Pavese (a chicken and vegetable broth with a poached egg, see page 30) and a chunky fish soup (Zuppa de Pesce, see page 29). These are a meal in themselves and ideal for a quick lunch or supper.

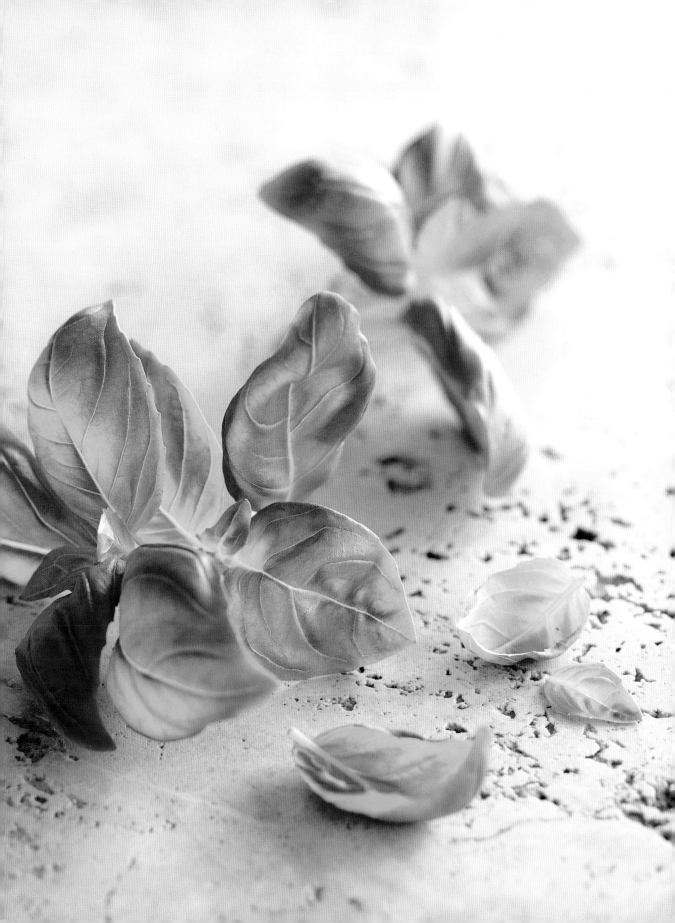

Fennel soup with roasted cherry tomatoes

SERVES 4

EASY Ⓥ

Syns per serving
Extra Easy: Free
Original: Free
Green: Free

Preparation time: 20 minutes
Cooking time: under 1 hour

low calorie cooking spray
2 medium onions, peeled and
finely chopped
1 garlic clove, finely chopped
2 fennel bulbs (about 450g/1lb in
total), trimmed and finely sliced
900ml/1½ pints vegetable stock
finely grated zest of ½ orange
200g/7oz fat free natural fromage frais
salt and freshly ground black pepper
200g/7oz cherry tomatoes on the vine
2 tbsp finely chopped dill or
fennel fronds

This popular summery Italian soup makes a great starter for any lunch or dinner party, and can be made well in advance. You then only have to roast the tomatoes before serving.

Spray a large, heavy-based saucepan with low calorie cooking spray. Add the onions and garlic, cover and cook over a very gentle heat for 10 minutes without colouring.

Add the fennel and cook gently for 10 minutes, stirring often, to bring out the full flavour of the fennel.

Add the stock and orange zest. Cover, bring to the boil and simmer gently for about 30 minutes or until the vegetables are tender.

Cool the soup a little, then purée in a liquidiser and pass through a sieve. Stir in the fromage frais and season to taste.

Meanwhile, preheat the oven to 200°C/Gas 6. Place the tomatoes on a non-stick baking sheet and cook in the oven for 15–20 minutes or until softened.

To serve, reheat the soup gently and ladle into shallow soup plates. Top each serving with some of the roasted cherry tomatoes and scatter over the dill or fennel fronds. This soup is delicious served hot or chilled.

Winter minestrone

SERVES 4

EASY Ⓥ ❄

Syns per serving
Extra Easy: Free
Green: Free
Original: 9 Syns

Preparation time: 20 minutes
Cooking time: 40–45 minutes

1 onion, peeled and finely chopped
150g/5oz swede, peeled and cut into bite-sized pieces
150g/5oz turnips, peeled and cut into bite-sized pieces
1 large carrot, peeled and cut into bite-sized pieces
2 celery sticks, roughly chopped
1 medium potato, peeled and cut into bite-sized pieces
2 garlic cloves, peeled and crushed
400g can chopped tomatoes
1 litre/1¾ pints vegetable stock
2 tsp finely chopped sage
50g/2oz short-shaped dried pasta or macaroni
400g can borlotti beans, drained and rinsed
4 tbsp finely chopped flat-leaf parsley
salt and freshly ground black pepper

Perfect for an autumnal or winter lunch, this warming and substantial soup is made using all of the winter root vegetables, but you can use whatever you have at hand.

Place the onion, swede, turnips, carrot, celery, potato and garlic in a large saucepan.

Add the tomatoes, stock and sage and bring to the boil, stirring occasionally. Reduce the heat to a simmer and cook the vegetables, partly covered, for 30–35 minutes, stirring in the pasta after 15 minutes and cook until the pasta and vegetables are tender.

Add the borlotti beans to the pan with the parsley, season well and remove from the heat.

Serve immediately.

Tuscan bean soup

SERVES 4

EASY (V) (✽)

Syns per serving
Extra Easy: Free
Green: Free
Original: 13 Syns

Preparation time: 20 minutes
Cooking time: under 45 minutes

2 celery sticks, finely sliced
1 leek, trimmed and finely sliced
1 large carrot, peeled and
finely chopped
600g/1lb 5oz curly kale, stems removed
and leaves roughly shredded
400g/14oz potatoes, peeled and
finely diced
1 level tsp tomato purée
2 bay leaves
4 thyme sprigs
1.5 litres/2½ pints vegetable stock
400g can cannellini beans, drained
and rinsed
400g can borlotti beans, drained
and rinsed
sea salt and freshly
ground black pepper
2 tbsp roughly chopped parsley

This hearty and healthy soup can be turned into a smooth broth by liquidising, if preferred.

Place a large saucepan over a low heat add the celery, leek and carrot. Stir-fry over a gentle heat for 10 minutes.

Add the kale, potatoes, tomato purée, bay leaves, thyme sprigs and stock and simmer, covered, for 30 minutes or until the vegetables are tender.

Mash one-third of the beans to a paste, add to the soup with the rest of the beans and cook for 3–4 minutes, stirring well.

Season well and scatter with chopped parsley before serving.

Zuppa de pesce

SERVES 4

EASY ✳ (if fish not previously frozen)

Syns per serving
Extra Easy: Free
Original: Free
Green: 22½ Syns

Preparation time: 15 minutes
Cooking time: under 25 minutes

1 bay leaf
1 large rosemary sprig
1 tbsp fennel seeds, coarsely crushed
1 fennel bulb, trimmed and chopped
3 large shallots, peeled and chopped
salt and freshly ground black pepper
400g can chopped cherry tomatoes
a strip of orange peel
800ml/28fl oz fish stock
1kg/2lb 4oz assorted firm-fleshed fish
fillets (cod, halibut, salmon or tuna),
skinned and cut into large pieces
500g/1lb 2oz raw tiger prawns, peeled
2 tbsp finely chopped flat-leaf parsley

The flavours of Italy are packed into this delicious and wholesome fish soup.

Wrap the bay leaf, rosemary and fennel seeds in a muslin bag to make a bouquet garni. Set aside until needed.

Place a large saucepan over a medium heat. Add the fennel and shallots and sauté for about 6 minutes until the fennel is tender. Season well.

Add the tomatoes with their juices, orange peel and fish stock. Add the bouquet garni and bring the mixture to a boil. Reduce the heat to medium-low, then cover and let the soup simmer for 10 minutes.

Add the fish and prawns to the mixture. Simmer for 4–5 minutes or until they are just cooked through.

Remove the bouquet garni and the orange peel, stir in the chopped parsley and check the seasoning. Serve immediately.

Zuppa alla pavese

To make a change, you can substitute turkey for the chicken in this delicious and hearty broth.

SERVES 4

EASY ✽ (without the poached egg)

Syns per serving
Extra Easy: Free
Original: Free
Green: 13 Syns

Preparation time: 15–20 minutes
Cooking time: under 40 minutes

low calorie cooking spray
6 spring onions, trimmed and
finely chopped
3 celery sticks, finely chopped
1 garlic clove, peeled and
finely chopped
150g/5oz courgettes, cut into
bite-sized cubes
300g/11oz carrots, peeled and cut into
bite-sized cubes
pared zest from 1 small lemon
1.5 litres/2½ pints chicken or
vegetable stock
3 cooked chicken breasts
(approximately 600g/1lb 5oz), skinned
and roughly shredded
50g/2oz spring greens, shredded
salt and freshly ground black pepper
4 medium eggs

Spray a large, heavy-based saucepan with low calorie cooking spray. Add the spring onions, celery and garlic and stir-fry for 2–3 minutes until softened but not coloured.

Add the courgette, carrots and lemon zest and stir-fry for 2–3 minutes.

Add the stock and bring to the boil. Reduce the heat to medium-low and simmer for 25 minutes, or until the carrots are tender.

Add the chicken and spring greens and cook for 5–6 minutes. Season to taste.

Meanwhile, bring a large saucepan of lightly salted water to a very gentle simmer. One by one, carefully crack each egg into a small bowl and slide into the simmering water. Cook them together for 2–3 minutes and then remove from the heat. Allow to stand in the water for 3–4 minutes.

Ladle the soup into warmed, shallow soup plates. Carefully remove the eggs from the saucepan with a slotted spoon and place a poached egg over each soup serving. Serve immediately.

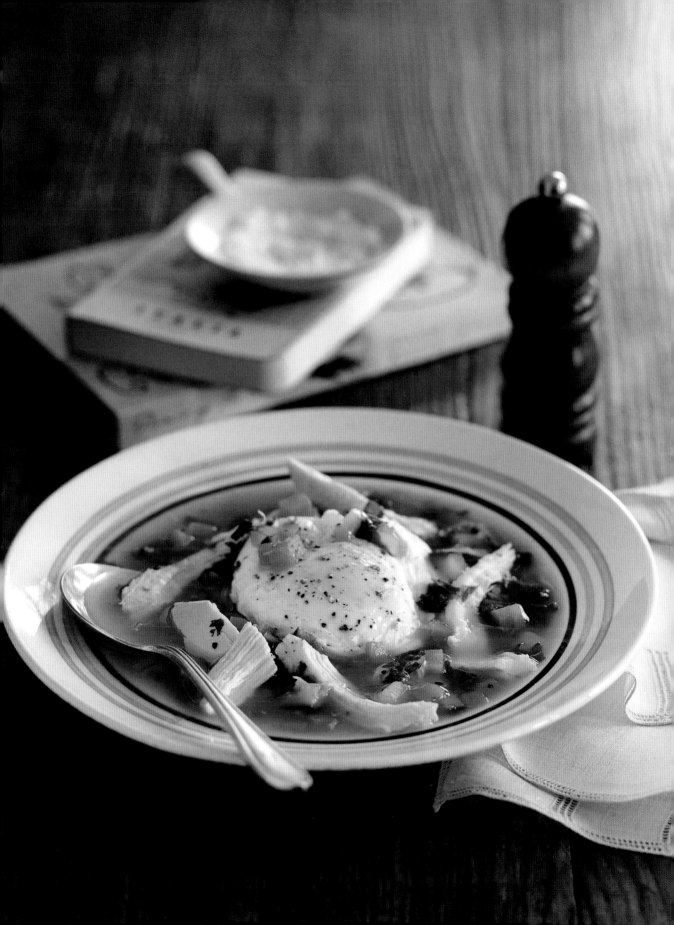

Tomato and basil bruschetta

Always try to use the ripest and most flavoursome tomatoes for this simple, but delicious Italian starter.

Spray the ciabatta slices with low calorie cooking spray and toast both sides on a hot griddle. Rub the toasted bread with the garlic.

Mix the tomatoes with the basil and season well.

Spoon the mixture onto the toasted bread and serve garnished with wild rocket.

Grilled peppers with garlic, chilli and parsley

SERVES 4

EASY (V) (❄)

Syns per serving
Extra Easy: Free
Original: Free
Green: Free

Preparation time: 10 minutes
Cooking time: 20 minutes

4 red peppers, deseeded and
cut into thick strips
4 yellow peppers, deseeded and
cut into thick strips
2 orange peppers, deseeded and
cut into thick strips
6 garlic cloves, peeled and
finely chopped
1–2 tsp dried red chilli flakes
juice of 1 large lemon
salt and freshly ground black pepper
4 tbsp finely chopped flat-leaf parsley

This piquant starter is perfect for summer entertaining as it can be made ahead of time and it's ideal for al fresco dining.

Place the pepper strips in a large roasting tin. Scatter over the garlic, red chilli flakes and half of the lemon juice and season well. Toss to coat the pepper strips in the seasonings.

Preheat the grill to medium-high. Place the peppers in a grill pan and cook on the top shelf for about 20 minutes, turning occasionally, until all peppers are soft and some are slightly charred.

Remove from the grill and place the peppers and any accumulated juices into a wide bowl or container. Add the remaining lemon juice and the chopped parsley and toss to mix well.

Serve them warm as a starter or you can chill them in the fridge for a few hours and then serve at room temperature.

Stuffed tomatoes with green rice

SERVES 4

WORTH THE EFFORT Ⓥ ❋

Syns per serving
Extra Easy: Free
Green: Free
Original: 2½ Syns

Preparation time: 15 minutes plus standing
Cooking time: 35–40 minutes

4 large, firm tomatoes (about 700g/ 1lb 9oz in total)
2 garlic cloves, peeled and crushed
50g/2oz dried risotto rice
6 tbsp finely chopped basil
2 spring onions, trimmed and finely chopped
salt and freshly ground black pepper

This classic Italian starter of stuffed, baked tomatoes also makes a great accompaniment to any chicken or fish dish as well being a main course dish in its own right.

Cut a slice off the top of each tomato and set aside to use as lids. Scoop out the pulp from the tomatoes and chop finely. Transfer to a large bowl with any of the tomato juices.

Stir in the garlic, rice, basil and spring onions and season well. Cover and leave to stand at room temperature for 1 hour, for the rice to soak up all the juices.

Preheat the oven to 180°C/Gas 4. Stuff the tomatoes with the rice mixture and transfer to a non-stick baking dish. Top with the reserved lids and bake the tomatoes in the oven for 35–40 minutes or until the tomatoes are soft and the rice is cooked through.

Serve warm or at room temperature.

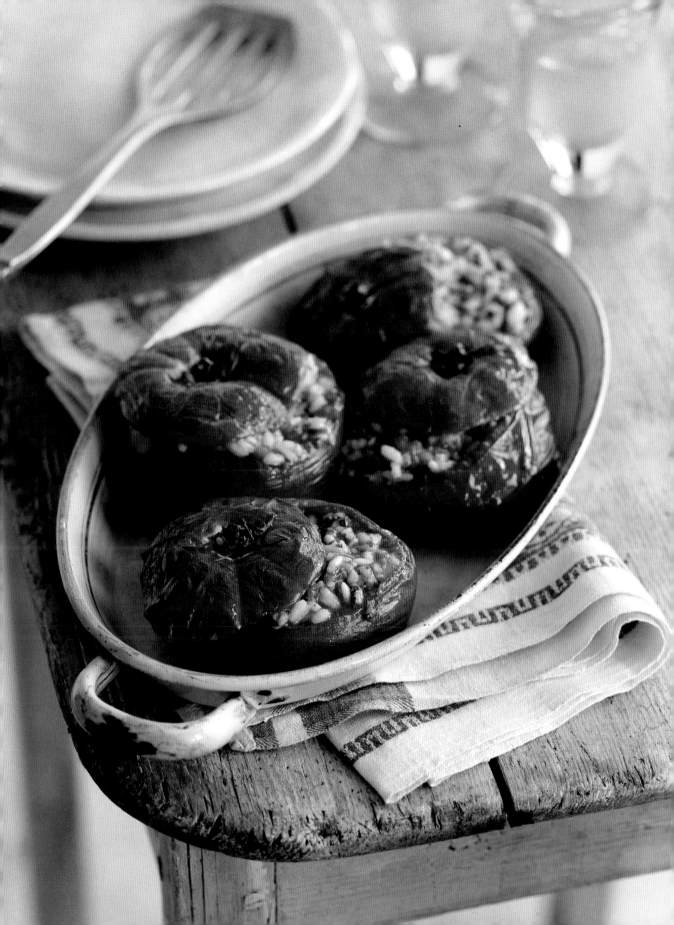

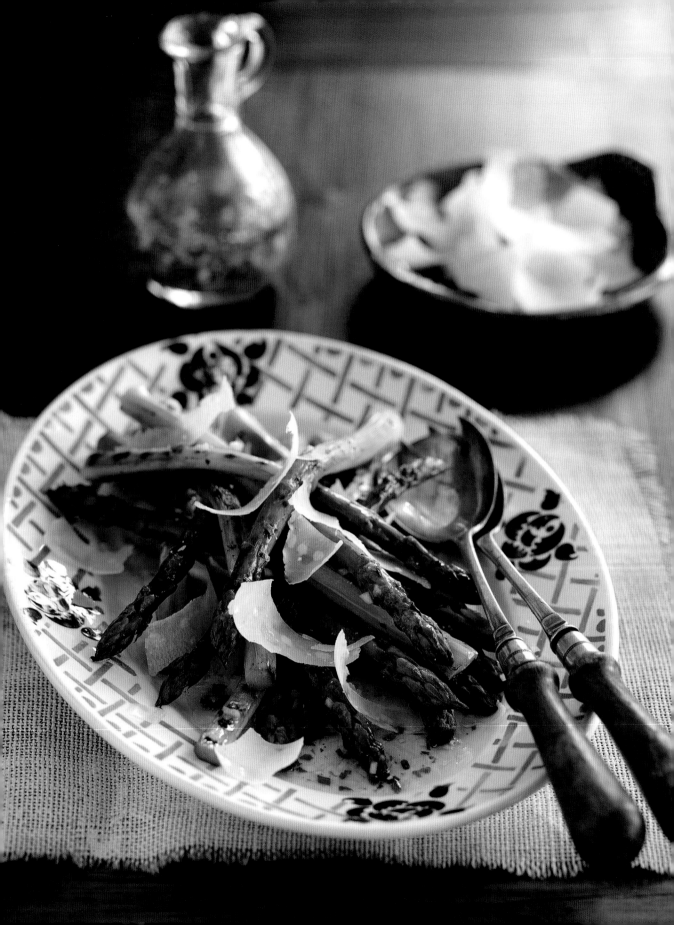

Char-grilled asparagus with Pecorino

SERVES 4

REALLY EASY

Syns per serving
Extra Easy: ½ Syn
Original: ½ Syn
Green: ½ Syn

Preparation time: 15 minutes
Cooking time: about 10 minutes

24 asparagus spears,
hard stalks removed
low calorie cooking spray
15g/½oz Pecorino cheese, shaved into
thin strips

FOR THE LEMON AND CHIVE DRESSING
juice of 1 lemon
200ml/7fl oz fat free vinaigrette
1 shallot, peeled and finely chopped
a small handful of chives, chopped
salt and freshly ground black pepper

This quick, easy and delicious starter can be made a couple of hours ahead of time and served at room temperature.

Bring a large saucepan of lightly salted water to the boil. Add the asparagus to the water and blanch for 1–2 minutes.

Using tongs or a slotted spoon, remove the asparagus from the boiling water and place immediately into a bowl of iced water, then drain.

Heat a non-stick griddle until very hot. Spray the asparagus with low calorie cooking spray and place onto the hot griddle. Cook in batches, for 2–3 minutes, turning occasionally, until nicely marked and browned on all sides.

To make the dressing, mix the lemon juice with the vinaigrette, chopped shallot and chives in a bowl and season to taste.

Transfer the asparagus to a serving plate or dish. Drizzle over the lemon and chive vinaigrette and sprinkle over the shaved Pecorino.

Suppli (baked risotto balls)

SERVES 4

WORTH THE EFFORT ✻

Syns per serving
Extra Easy: 4 Syns
Green: 4 Syns
Original: 22 Syns

Preparation time: 1 hour plus chilling
Cooking time: 12–15 minutes

25g/1oz dried porcini mushrooms
low calorie cooking spray
2 leeks, trimmed and finely chopped
200g/7oz mixed mushrooms, roughly chopped
salt and freshly ground black pepper
1 onion, peeled and finely chopped
1 tsp dried thyme
1 bay leaf
400g/14oz dried risotto rice
2 litres/3½ pints boiling hot vegetable stock
6 tbsp finely chopped flat-leaf parsley
4 level tbsp finely grated Parmesan cheese
2 large eggs
50g/2oz dried wholemeal breadcrumbs
salad leaves, to serve

This starter is perfect for entertaining as it can be prepared up to a day in advance and quickly cooked when ready to serve.

Soak the dried mushrooms in a bowl with 300ml/ 11fl oz of hot water for 15 minutes. Drain, reserve the liquid and chop the mushrooms. Set aside.

Spray a large non-stick frying pan with low calorie cooking spray, add the leeks and cook over a gentle heat for 2–3 minutes. Add the fresh mushrooms and cook for 5–6 minutes. Season to taste, transfer to a bowl and set aside.

Wipe out the frying pan and return to the heat. Add the onion, thyme and bay leaf and cook, stirring, for a few minutes. Add the rice and cook for 1 minute, stirring so all the grains are well coated. Pour the mushroom soaking liquid over the rice and simmer, stirring, until it has been absorbed. Add the rehydrated mushrooms.

Bring the stock to a simmer and add to the pan, a ladleful at a time, stirring. Allow each ladleful to be absorbed before adding the next. Add the sautéed mushrooms, parsley and half of the Parmesan cheese. Stir well. Season to taste and spread onto a non-stick tray and leave to cool.

Whisk the eggs in a bowl. Mix the remaining Parmesan with the breadcrumbs. Make 20 balls of the risotto, dip in the egg and then in the breadcrumbs. Put on a baking sheet lined with baking parchment and chill for at least 1 hour.

Preheat the oven to 200°C/Gas 6. Spray the balls with low calorie cooking spray and bake for 12–15 minutes. Serve warm with the salad leaves.

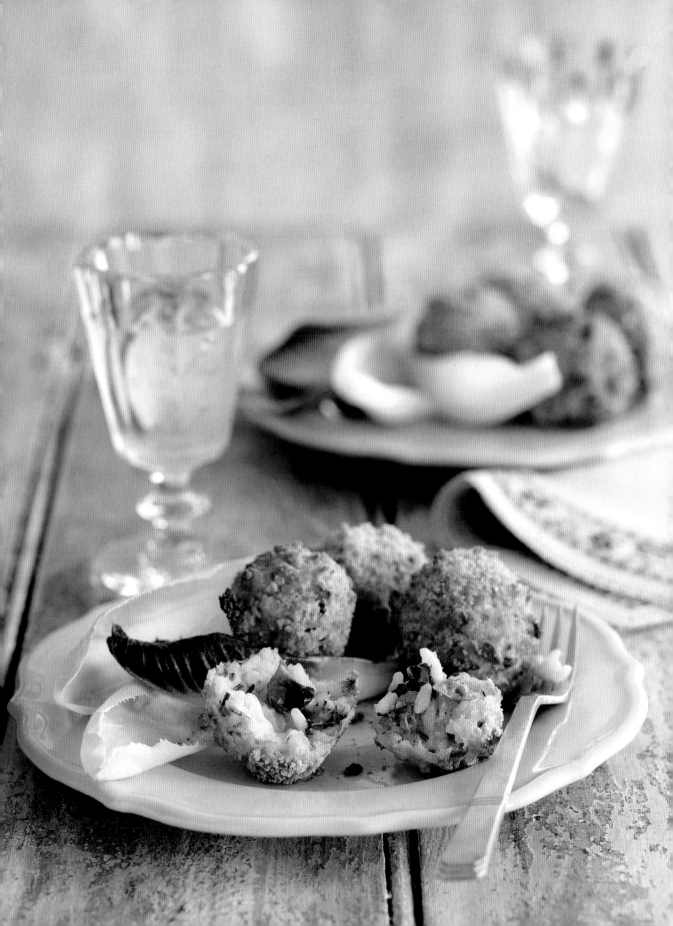

Baked stuffed mushrooms

SERVES 4

EASY Ⓥ ❄

Syns per serving
Extra Easy: Free
Original: Free
Green: Free

Preparation time: 20 minutes
Cooking time: 15–20 minutes

8 large cap mushrooms
low calorie cooking spray
4 spring onions, trimmed and
finely sliced
salt and freshly ground black pepper
2 garlic cloves, peeled and crushed
100g/3½oz quark
1 tbsp finely grated lemon zest
1 tbsp finely chopped oregano
2 tbsp finely chopped flat-leaf parsley
salad leaves, to serve

Always use fresh, large, firm mushrooms for this dish for the best possible texture and flavour.

Preheat the oven to 190°C/Gas 5. Remove the stalks from the mushrooms and finely chop them.

Spray a frying pan with low calorie cooking spray, add the mushroom stalks and spring onions and stir-fry over a high heat for 4–5 minutes. Season well and transfer to a bowl with the garlic, quark, lemon zest and chopped herbs.

Place the mushroom caps gill side up on a baking sheet lined with non-stick baking parchment. Divide the stuffing among the caps and bake in the oven for 15–20 minutes.

Serve the mushrooms hot or warm with a mixture of salad leaves.

Garlic prawns

SERVES 4

EASY

Syns per serving
Extra Easy: Free
Original: Free
Green: 2 Syns

Preparation time: 15 minutes
Cooking time: 3–4 minutes

6 garlic cloves, peeled and
finely chopped
finely grated zest and juice of 1 lemon
1 tsp dried red chilli flakes
1 mild red chilli, deseeded and
finely diced
4 tbsp finely chopped parsley
24 raw tiger prawns, peeled but
with tails left on
salt
a handful of wild rocketleaves,
to serve

Turn this delicious and moreish starter into a main meal by tossing it with cooked pasta.

Place the garlic, lemon zest and juice, dried chilli flakes, red chilli and parsley in a ceramic bowl. Add the prawns to the garlic mixture. Toss to mix well and season with salt.

Heat a large non-stick frying pan until it is very hot. Add the prawn mixture and stir-fry for 3–4 minutes or until the prawns turn pink and are cooked through. Remove from the heat.

Line four serving plates with the rocket leaves and top with the warm prawn mixture. You can serve these prawns immediately or at room temperature, if preferred.

Seafood antipasto

SERVES 4

WORTH THE EFFORT

Syns per serving
Extra Easy: Free
Original: Free
Green: 10½ Syns

Preparation time: 30 minutes
plus chilling
Cooking time: under 25 minutes

500g/1lb 2oz mussels, cleaned
300g/11oz clams, cleaned
1 onion, peeled and quartered
1 bay leaf
300g/11oz small squid, cleaned and
cut into 2.5cm/1in rounds
500g/1lb 2oz raw, peeled king prawns
juice of 2 lemons
2 garlic cloves, peeled and
finely chopped
4 tbsp fat free vinaigrette
salt and freshly ground black pepper
2 celery sticks, thinly sliced
1 carrot, peeled and finely diced
1 red pepper, deseeded and
finely diced
3 spring onions, trimmed and
thinly sliced

You can vary the seafood in this dish to suit your needs. It makes a great light lunch or supper when tossed with cooked rice or pasta.

Place the mussels and clams in a large saucepan with 100ml/3½fl oz of water. Cover and bring to the boil over a high heat. Cook, shaking the pan from time to time, for 4–5 minutes or until all the shells have opened, discarding any that remain closed. Remove the flesh from the shells and place in a large bowl.

Return the pan with the cooking liquid to a high heat and add 400ml/14fl oz of water, the onion and bay leaf and bring to the boil.

Add the squid and prawns to the stock and cook for 2–3 minutes or until the prawns turn pink. Remove with a slotted spoon and add to the mussels and clams.

Boil the liquid in the pan until reduced to about 60ml/2fl oz, remove from the heat and stir in the lemon juice, garlic and vinaigrette. Season well and pour over the seafood mixture.

Stir in the celery, carrot, red pepper and spring onions and toss to mix well. Cover and chill for 1–2 hours before serving.

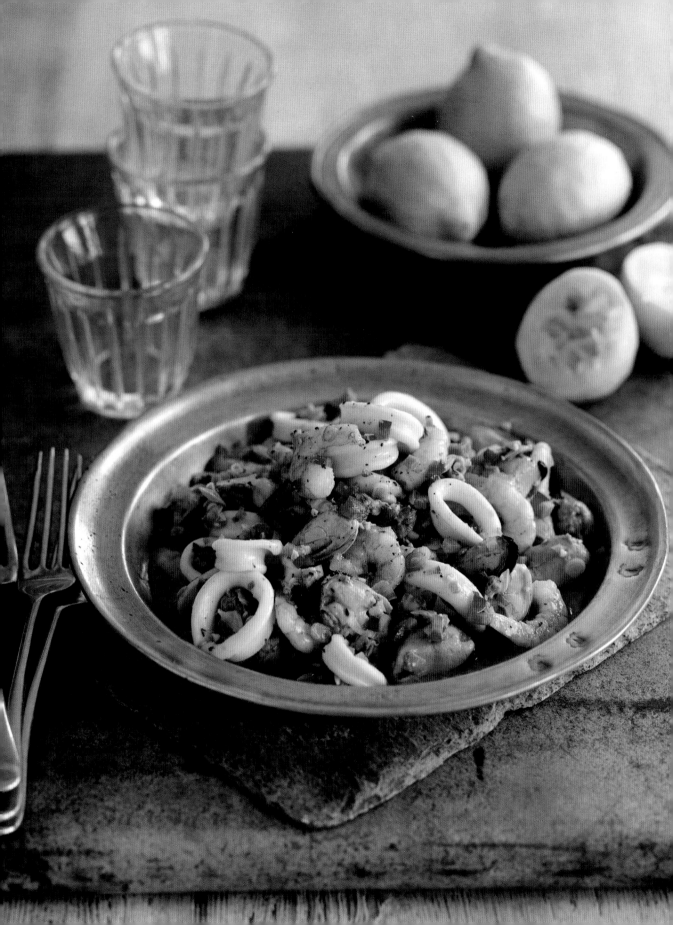

Marinated grilled sardines

SERVES 4

EASY

Syns per serving
Extra Easy: Free
Original: Free
Green: 35 Syns

Preparation time: 10 minutes
plus marinating
Cooking time: 12–15 minutes

12 sardines, cleaned and
heads removed
2 tbsp white wine vinegar
2 garlic cloves, peeled and crushed
1 red chilli, deseeded and
finely chopped
2 tbsp finely chopped flat-leaf parsley
salt
crisp salad leaves, to serve
lemon wedges, to serve

You can cook these sardines on a barbecue in the summer for extra flavour. You can also substitute four mackerel for the sardines, if desired.

Place the sardines in a shallow, ceramic dish in a single layer.

Mix the vinegar, garlic, red chilli and parsley together and spoon this mixture over the sardines. Season with salt, cover and marinate in the fridge for 1 hour, turning once.

Preheat the grill to medium-high. Remove the sardines from the marinade and place on a grill rack. Drizzle with the marinade from the dish and cook under the grill for 12–15 minutes, turning once, or until the fish is cooked through and slightly charred at the edges.

Serve hot on crisp salad leaves with lemon wedges to squeeze over.

Tuna carpaccio

SERVES 4

WORTH THE EFFORT

Syns per serving
Extra Easy: Free
Original: Free
Green: 8½ Syns

Preparation time: 10 minutes
plus chilling
Cooking time: under 5 minutes

500g/1lb 2oz tuna loin, trimmed
low calorie cooking spray
4 tbsp crushed black peppercorns
2 tsp dried red chilli flakes
50g/2oz wild rocket leaves
1 large cucumber, halved, deseeded
and finely sliced
juice of 1 large lemon
salt and freshly ground black pepper

When buying the tuna for this dish, choose the freshest and best quality tuna from your fishmonger or the fish counter of your local supermarket.

Spray the tuna with low calorie cooking spray and roll in the crushed pepper and chilli flakes.

Heat a dry non-stick pan over a high heat until very hot and sear the tuna for 2 minutes on each side. (The tuna should still be pink in the middle.)

Place the tuna on a plate and chill in the fridge for 30 minutes. Then remove from the fridge and slice thinly.

Arrange the rocket leaves and cucumber slices on serving plates. Squeeze over the lemon juice and season to taste. Divide the tuna slices between the plates and serve immediately.

Pancetta and vegetable spiedini

SERVES 4

EASY (❄)

Syns per serving
Extra Easy: 2 Syns
Original: 2 Syns
Green: 4 Syns

Preparation time: 15 minutes
Cooking time: 8–10 minutes

8 medium mushrooms, quartered
1 large red onion, peeled and
cut into wedges
1 courgette, sliced into thick rounds
8 thin slices lean pancetta
salt and freshly ground black pepper
1 tbsp finely chopped rosemary
low calorie cooking spray
lemon wedges, to serve

These tasty skewers can be prepared a couple of hours ahead and chilled in the fridge until ready to cook and serve.

Preheat the grill to medium-high.

Thread the vegetables and the pancetta slices alternately between four metal or pre-soaked bamboo skewers, season well and sprinkle over the chopped rosemary.

Spray with low calorie cooking spray, place under the grill and cook for 8–10 minutes, turning occasionally, or until the vegetables have softened and the pancetta is crisp.

Remove from the heat and serve with lemon wedges to squeeze over.

Bresaola and rocket rolls

SERVES 4 (makes 16)

REALLY EASY

Syns per serving
Extra Easy: 1 Syn
Original: 1 Syn
Green: 4 Syns

Preparation time: 10 minutes
Cooking time: none

200g/7oz quark
2 garlic cloves, peeled and crushed
4 tbsp very finely chopped parsley
finely grated zest and juice of 1 lemon
salt and freshly ground black pepper
16 very thin slices bresaola
100g/3½oz wild rocket leaves
2–3 tbsp balsamic vinegar, to serve
lemon wedges, to serve

Bresaola is Italian cured dried beef and it can be found on the delicatessen counter of larger supermarkets and stores. You can substitute the beef with Parma ham in this recipe, if wished.

Mix together the quark, garlic, parsley and lemon zest and juice in a bowl until smooth. Season well with salt and pepper.

Lay the bresaola on a large board and spread the quark mixture over the meat slices.

Place a few rocket leaves across the middle of each slice.

Roll up each slice neatly and place on a serving platter. Serve drizzled with the balsamic vinegar and the lemon wedges to squeeze over.

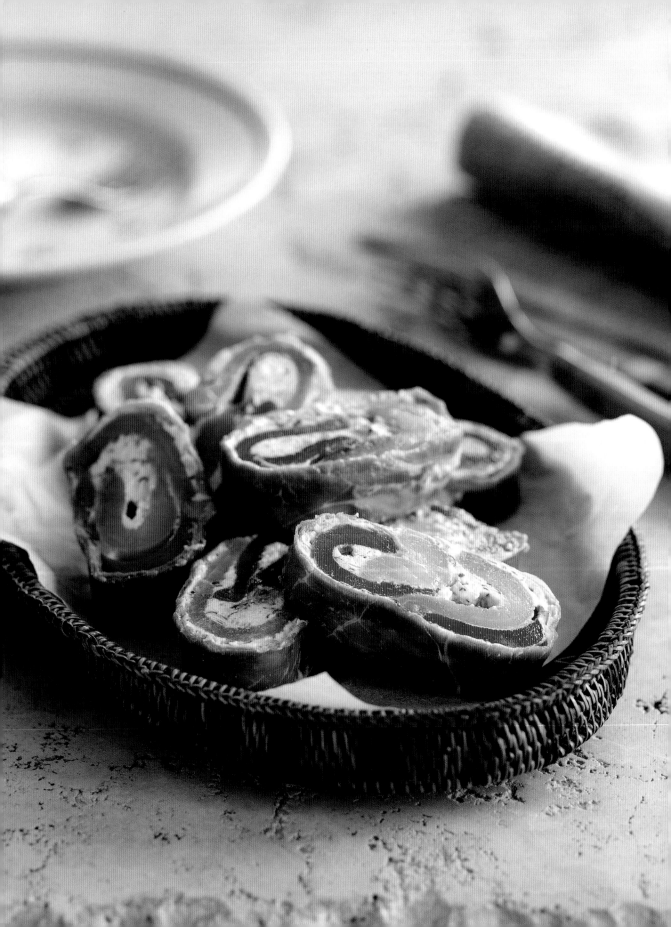

Prosciutto and grilled pepper pinwheels

These tasty pinwheels are an impressive starter and worth the effort for any lunch or dinner party.

SERVES 4 (makes about 20)

WORTH THE EFFORT

Syns per serving
Extra Easy: 1½ Syns
Original: 1½ Syns
Green: 4½ Syns

Preparation time: 25 minutes plus chilling
Cooking time: none

1 red pepper, deseeded and cut into quarters
1 yellow pepper, deseeded and cut into quarters
1 orange pepper, deseeded and cut into quarters
250g/9oz quark
2 garlic cloves, peeled and crushed
2 tbsp finely chopped basil
2 spring onions, trimmed and finely chopped
salt and freshly ground black pepper
12 thin slices lean prosciutto

Preheat the grill to high. Grill the peppers, skin side up, for 8–10 minutes, until the skin is blistered and lightly charred. Transfer to a plastic bag and allow to cool. When cool, carefully peel off the skins.

In a bowl, mix together the quark, garlic, basil and spring onions and season well.

Lay the prosciutto slices on a clean work surface, slightly overlapping each other.

Place the pepper pieces onto the prosciutto slices in a single layer and trim the prosciutto to the same size, to form a neat rectangle. Remove the pepper pieces and spread half of the quark mixture onto the prosciutto slices. Top with the pepper slices and spread the remaining quark mixture over them.

Roll up tightly from the short end, to form a neat cylinder. Wrap in cling film and chill in the fridge for 3–4 hours (or overnight if time permits).

To serve, remove the cling film and slice into 1.5cm/½in rounds or pinwheels and serve immediately.

Grilled beef skewers with salsa verde

SERVES 4

EASY ❄

Syns per serving
Extra Easy: Free
Original: Free
Green: 13 Syns

Preparation time: 20 minutes
plus marinating
Cooking time: 8–10 minutes

FOR THE SKEWERS
800g/1lb 12oz lean beef, all visible fat
removed and cut into bite-sized pieces
2 red peppers, deseeded and
cut into bite-sized pieces
2 red onions, peeled and cut into bite-
sized wedges
juice of 1 lemon
1 tsp paprika
100g/3½oz fat free natural yogurt
chopped parsley, to serve

FOR THE SALSA VERDE
40g/1½oz flat-leaf parsley
20g/¾oz basil
25g/1oz mint
4 tbsp red wine vinegar
2 garlic cloves, peeled and crushed
2 canned anchovy fillets in oil,
drained and chopped
2 tbsp capers, rinsed
120ml/4½fl oz fat free vinaigrette,
or more if required
salt and freshly ground black pepper

Salsa verde is a classic Italian green sauce and it can be served with any grilled fish, chicken or meat dish.

Place the beef in a ceramic bowl with the peppers and onions.

In a separate bowl, mix together the lemon juice, paprika and yogurt and stir into the beef and pepper mixture. Toss well to coat evenly and season to taste. Marinate for 6–8 hours (or overnight if time permits).

Meanwhile, make the salsa verde by placing the herbs and vinegar in a food processor and pulse until you have a coarse paste. Add the garlic, anchovies and half of the capers and pulse again.

Gradually add the vinaigrette with the motor running, but try not to process to too fine a purée. Transfer to a bowl. Season with freshly ground black pepper and the rest of the capers, and set aside, covered, until needed. Use within 24 hours.

When you're ready to eat, preheat the grill to hot. Thread the beef chunks, pepper pieces and onion wedges alternately onto eight metal or pre-soaked bamboo skewers and place under the grill. Cook for 8–10 minutes, turning once, or until the beef is cooked through and the vegetables are tender. Sprinkle with chopped parsley and serve immediately with the salsa verde spooned over.

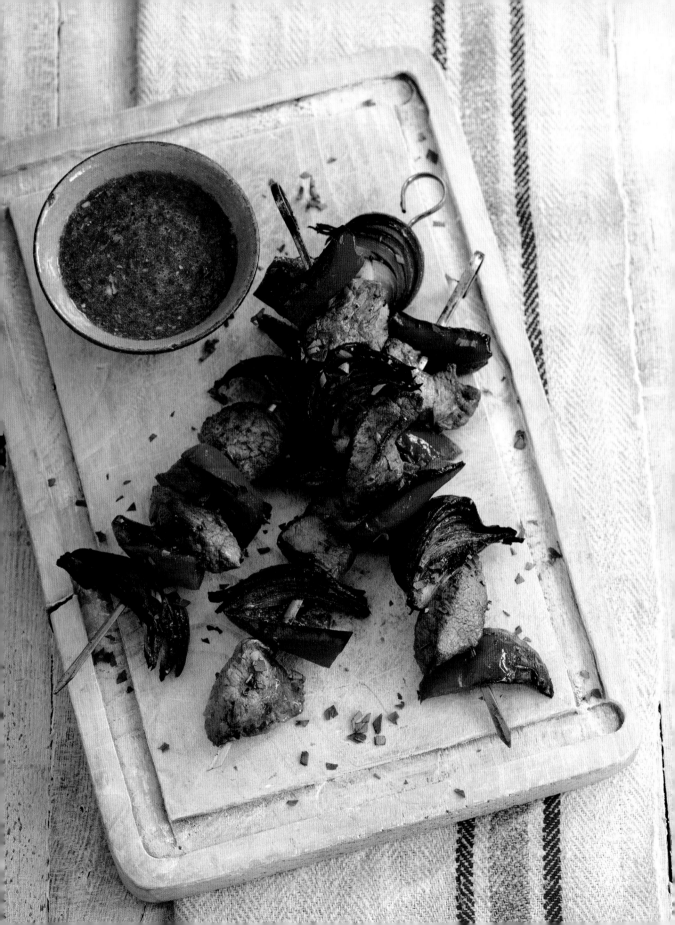

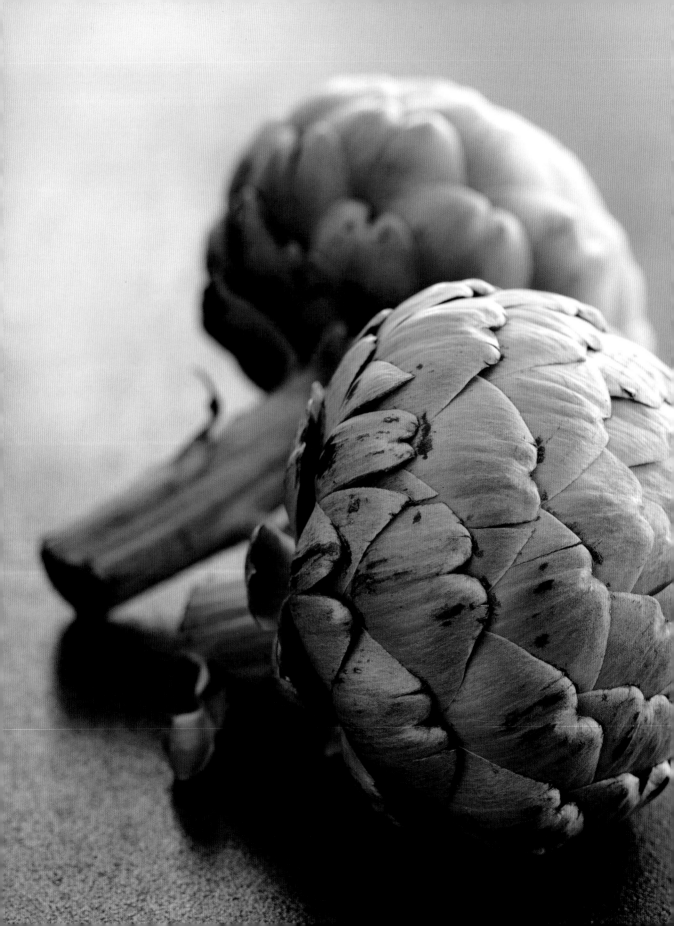

Chapter 2

Salads and snacks

You can always expect a taste sensation in an Italian salad, whether it's from an unusual marriage of ingredients, as in our Gorgonzola, Pear and Grape Salad (see page 55), Panzanella, a classic summer salad of bread and tomatoes (see page 62), or from a tangy dressing, made with balsamic vinegar or capers. Herbs and vegetables give colour and flavour to a traditional frittata (a set omelette, served just warm): try our Ham and Red Pepper Frittata on page 69. And Italians love finger food, such as crudités (vegetable sticks) with a dip, or herby chicken 'nuggets' or crostini – crisp, garlicky toast with a savoury topping.

Insalata caprese

SERVES 4

REALLY EASY Ⓥ

Syns per serving
Extra Easy: 2½ Syns
Original: 2½ Syns
Green: 2½ Syns

Preparation time: 5–10 minutes
Cooking time: none

4 ripe tomatoes
110g/4oz reduced fat mozzarella cheese
a large handful of basil leaves
juice of 1 lemon
salt and freshly ground black pepper

The flavours in this simple, classic Italian salad of tomatoes, basil and mozzarella come from using the freshest and best ingredients you can get your hands on.

Slice the tomatoes and arrange on the base of a serving platter.

Slice the mozzarella thinly and arrange over the tomatoes on the plate.

Scatter over the basil leaves and then drizzle over the lemon juice.

Season well, cover and allow to rest at room temperature for 30–60 minutes to allow the flavours to mingle before serving.

Gorgonzola, pear and grape salad

This salad is a wonderful combination of flavours, colours and textures.

SERVES 4

REALLY EASY (V)

Syns per serving
Extra Easy: 4½ Syns
Original: 4½ Syns
Green: 4½ Syns

Preparation time: 10 minutes
Cooking time: none

4 ripe pears
50g/2oz baby spinach leaves
50g/2oz red seedless grapes
50g/2oz green seedless grapes
110g/4oz gorgonzola cheese
200ml/7fl oz fat free vinaigrette
salt and freshly ground black pepper

Peel, quarter and core the pears and then cut them into thin wedges.

Divide the spinach between four serving plates and top with the pears.

Scatter over the grapes and crumble over the gorgonzola cheese.

Drizzle over the vinaigrette, season well and serve immediately.

Roasted balsamic baby onion salad

SERVES 4

WORTH THE EFFORT Ⓥ

Syns per serving
Extra Easy: Free
Original: Free
Green: Free

Preparation time: about 15 minutes plus marinating
Cooking time: about 1 hour

400g/14oz baby onions (also known as pearl onions or pickling onions), unpeeled
150ml/5fl oz balsamic vinegar
1 tbsp artificial sweetener
100g/3½oz mixed salad leaves
salt and freshly ground black pepper

This Sicilian-inspired salad is great for quick entertaining and perfect for a hot summer's day – just toss the onions with the salad leaves and serve.

Preheat the oven to 160°C/Gas 3.

Place the onions on a non-stick baking tray and bake for 1 hour. Remove from the oven and when cool enough to handle, trim the stems from the onions and peel away the skins.

Place the onions in a 1 litre/1¾ pint sterilised jar. Mix the vinegar with 150ml/5fl oz of water and the sweetener until well combined and pour this over the onions. Shake to mix well, seal the jar and place in the fridge to marinate overnight. (They can be left to marinate for 2–3 days.)

When ready to serve, place the salad leaves in a wide serving bowl. Drain the onions and scatter over the leaves. Season well, toss to combine and serve immediately.

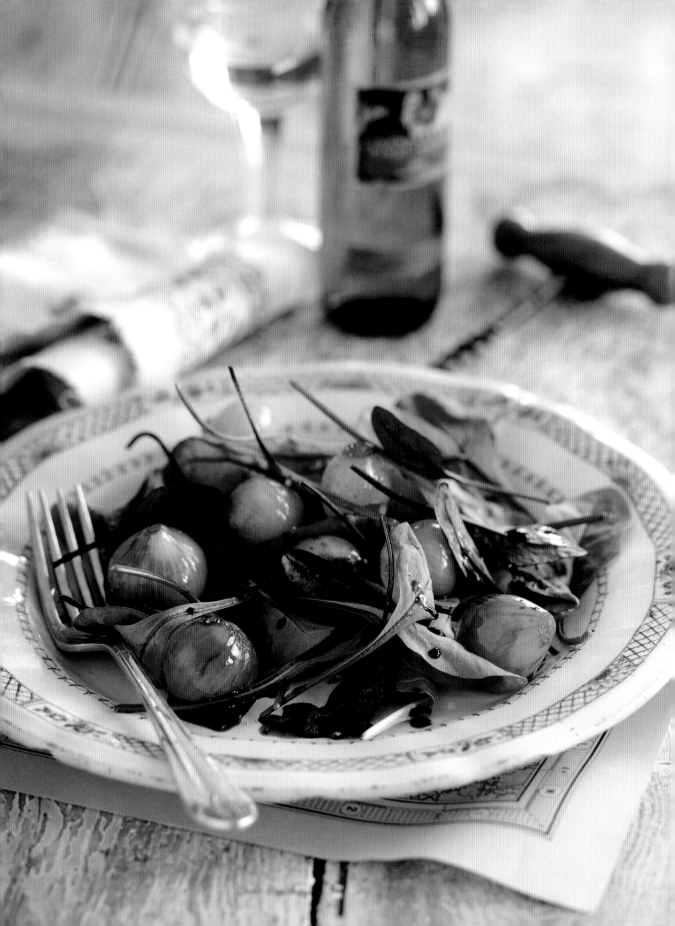

Caponata

SERVES 4

EASY Ⓥ ❄

Syns per serving
Extra Easy: Free
Original: Free
Green: Free

Preparation time: 15 minutes
Cooking time: under 40 minutes

4 medium aubergines,
cut into 2cm/¾in cubes
1 onion, peeled and roughly chopped
2 celery sticks, roughly chopped
2 red peppers, deseeded and
roughly chopped
400g can chopped tomatoes
3 tbsp rinsed and chopped capers
2 tbsp red wine vinegar
1 tbsp artificial sweetener, or to taste
a small handful of flat-leaf parsley,
chopped

There are dozens of variations of this delectable aubergine and pepper dish from Sicily. It is usually served as an antipasto, but is equally good with fish or steak.

Place the aubergines, onion, celery, red peppers and tomatoes in a saucepan and bring to the boil.

Reduce the heat to low, cover and cook gently for 20–25 minutes, stirring occasionally. Add the capers and stir to mix well.

In a separate bowl, mix together the red wine vinegar and sweetener. Add this to the vegetables in the pan and cook for 10 minutes.

Transfer to a large bowl, add the chopped parsley and mix well. Serve hot or at room temperature with crudités, or over wholemeal crostini (see Chicken Liver Crostini, page 000) (3 Syns per 25g/1oz) or cooked pasta (1½ Syns per 25g/1oz cooked on Original).

Griddled aubergine salad

SERVES 4

WORTH THE EFFORT (V)

Syns per serving
Extra Easy: Free
Original: Free
Green: Free

Preparation time: 10 minutes
plus resting
Cooking time: 15–20 minutes

2 medium aubergines (about
500g/1lb 2oz in total)
low calorie cooking spray

FOR THE DRESSING
finely grated zest and juice of
1 large lemon
2 tbsp balsamic vinegar
1 tsp artificial sweetener
1 tsp crushed dried
red chilli flakes (optional)
4 tbsp roughly chopped mint
salt and freshly ground black pepper

The secret of this very simple dish is the perfect cooking of the aubergine on a hot, hot griddle.

Make the dressing by placing the lemon zest and juice in a bowl with the balsamic vinegar, sweetener and chilli flakes, if using, and whisk well. Stir in half of the chopped mint. Season well and set aside.

Heat a non-stick ridged griddle until hot. Cut each aubergine into 8–10 thin slices and lightly spray with low calorie cooking spray. Cook the aubergine, in batches, on the hot griddle for 2–3 minutes on each side until lightly browned and lightly charred at the edges.

Arrange the aubergine slices on a large platter and spoon the dressing over the top. Cover and set aside for 30 minutes to let the aubergines absorb the dressing.

Sprinkle with the remaining mint before serving.

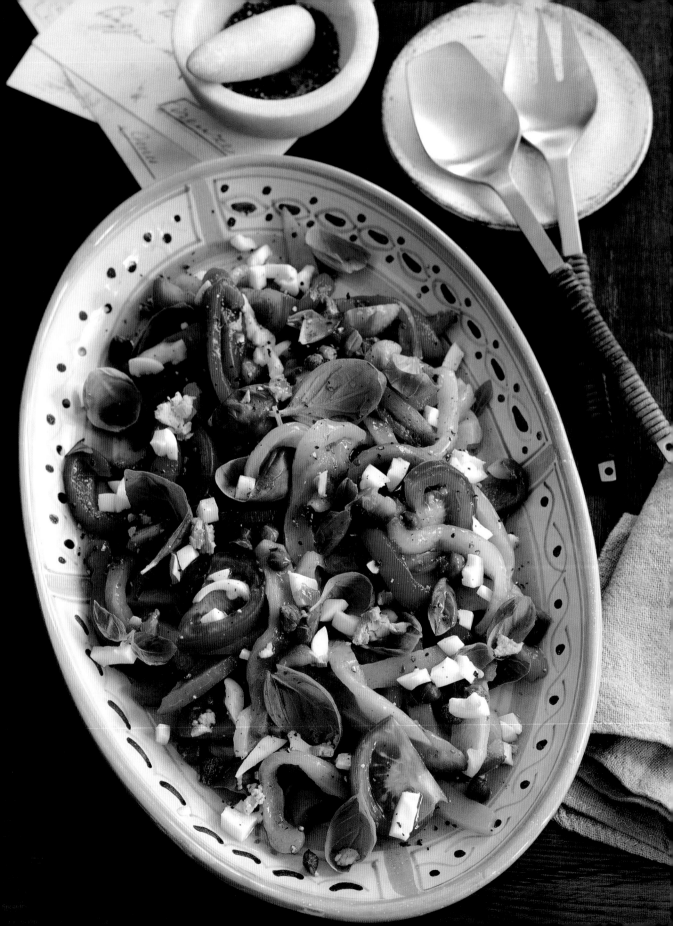

Mixed pepper salad with capers

SERVES 4

EASY (V)

Syns per serving
Extra Easy: Free
Original: Free
Green: Free

Preparation time: 5 minutes
Cooking time: 8–10 minutes

5 mixed peppers (green, red and
yellow), halved and deseeded
4 ripe plum tomatoes
2 tbsp fat free vinaigrette
2 tbsp red wine vinegar
2 tbsp capers, rinsed
2 large eggs, hard-boiled, peeled and
roughly chopped
a small bunch of basil, roughly torn
salt and freshly ground black pepper

This delicious mixed pepper salad gets its flavour and sweetness from grilling the peppers. It also makes a terrific accompaniment to any meat or fish dish.

Preheat the grill to high. Place the peppers skin side up on a grill rack and cook for 8–10 minutes or until the skin is charred. Transfer to a plastic bag and allow to cool. When cool, peel off the skins and cut the peppers into thick strips.

Cut the tomatoes into wedges and put them into a shallow serving dish.

Mix the vinaigrette and red wine vinegar together and pour over the tomatoes and peppers.

Scatter over the capers, chopped eggs and basil. Season well and serve at room temperature.

Panzanella

SERVES 4

EASY Ⓥ

Syns per serving
Extra Easy: 3 Syns
Original: 3 Syns
Green: 3 Syns

Preparation time: 15 minutes
Cooking time: none

2 tbsp red wine vinegar
2 garlic cloves, peeled and crushed
150ml/5fl oz fat free vinaigrette
1 small red onion, peeled, halved and
thinly sliced
500g/1lb 2oz ripe plum tomatoes,
cut into wedges
salt and freshly ground black pepper
4 slices wholemeal bread (from
a small 400g loaf)
a small handful of basil, torn,
to garnish
2 tbsp capers, rinsed, to garnish

This 'poor man's' tomato and bread salad is really tasty and benefits from being prepared ahead of time.

Mix the vinegar, garlic and vinaigrette together in a small bowl.

Place the onion and tomatoes in a wide ceramic salad bowl. Pour over the vinegar mixture, season well and toss to mix.

Cut the bread into 2.5cm/1in pieces and stir into the salad.

Cover the salad and leave it at room temperature for 2–3 hours for the flavours to mingle.

Just before serving, scatter over the basil and capers, toss to mix well and serve.

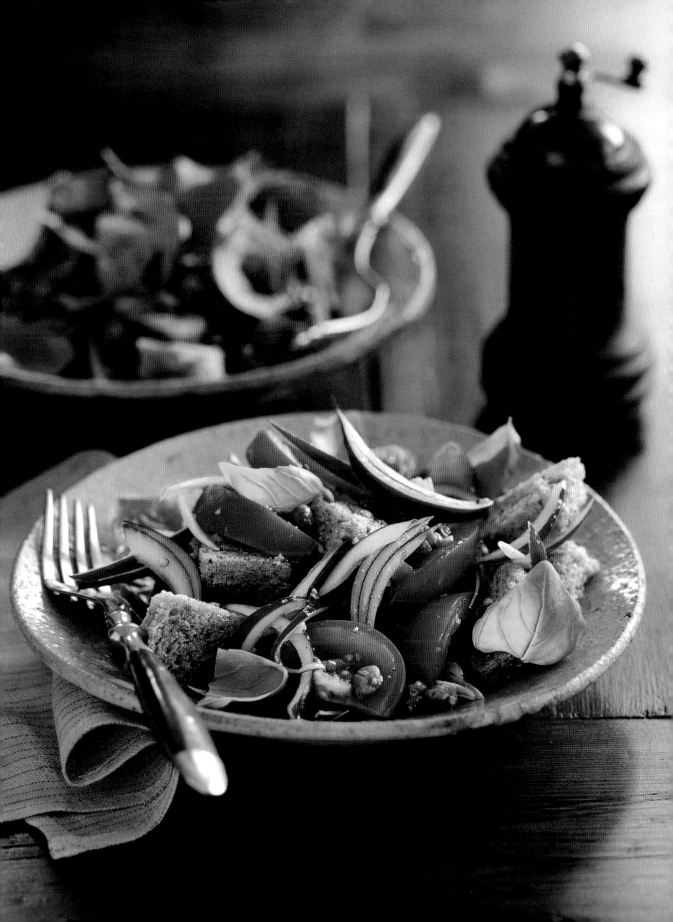

Prawn and green bean salad

In this salad, fresh green beans and raw prawns are quickly cooked and tossed together with roasted red peppers in a lemony dressing.

SERVES 4

EASY

Syns per serving
Extra Easy: Free
Original: Free
Green: 4 Syns

Preparation time: 10 minutes
Cooking time: under 10 minutes

300g/11oz fine green beans,
trimmed and halved
400g/14oz raw, peeled tiger prawns
100g/3½oz bottled roasted red peppers
in brine, drained and thickly sliced

FOR THE DRESSING
1 garlic clove, peeled and crushed
200ml/7fl oz fat free vinaigrette
juice of 1 lemon
1 shallot, peeled and finely diced
2 tbsp very finely chopped
flat-leaf parsley
salt and freshly ground black pepper

Bring a large pan of lightly salted water to the boil. Add the beans and blanch for 1–2 minutes, remove with a slotted spoon and plunge into a bowl of iced water. Drain well.

Add the prawns to the pan of boiling water and cook for 2–3 minutes or until they turn pink and are cooked through. Drain and transfer to a wide salad bowl with the beans and peppers.

Mix all the dressing ingredients together in a bowl and season well. Pour over the salad, toss gently to mix well and serve immediately.

Parma ham, melon and rocket salad

SERVES 4

REALLY EASY

Syns per serving
Extra Easy: 1 Syn
Original: 1 Syn
Green: 4 Syns

Preparation time: 10 minutes
Cooking time: none

1 cantaloupe melon
50g/2oz wild rocket leaves
8 thin slices lean Parma ham
freshly ground black pepper

FOR THE DRESSING
1 red chilli, deseeded and very finely chopped
1 tsp dried oregano
juice of ½ orange

Sun-sweetened melons, pungent rocket leaves and the saltiness of the Parma ham come together in this favourite summer salad.

Halve the melon and scoop out the seeds. Using a sharp knife, peel away the skin and cut the melon flesh into thin wedges or bite-sized pieces.

Arrange the rocket on four serving plates and divide the melon between them. Top each serving with two slices of the ham.

To make the dressing, mix together the red chilli, oregano and orange juice in a small bowl and drizzle over the salad.

Season with freshly ground black pepper and serve immediately.

Fig and Parma ham salad

SERVES 4

EASY

Syns per serving
Extra Easy: 1½ Syns
Original: 1½ Syns
Green: 6 Syns

Preparation time: 5 minutes
Cooking time: none

4 large or 8 small fresh ripe figs
50g/2oz wild rocket leaves
12 thin slices lean Parma ham
freshly ground black pepper
4 tbsp aged balsamic vinegar
very thin shavings of Parmesan cheese,
to garnish (optional)

The combination of salty Parma ham and the yielding soft sweet figs is an all-time Italian classic.

Take each fig and stand it upright on a clean work surface. Make two cuts across each fig, not quite quartering it, but keeping it intact at the base. Ease the figs open by pressing gently at the bottom.

Place the rocket on a serving plate. Arrange the Parma ham on the leaves and place the figs on the top. Season with freshly ground black pepper and then drizzle over the balsamic vinegar.

Serve garnished with the Parmesan shavings (3 Syns per 15g/½oz), if using.

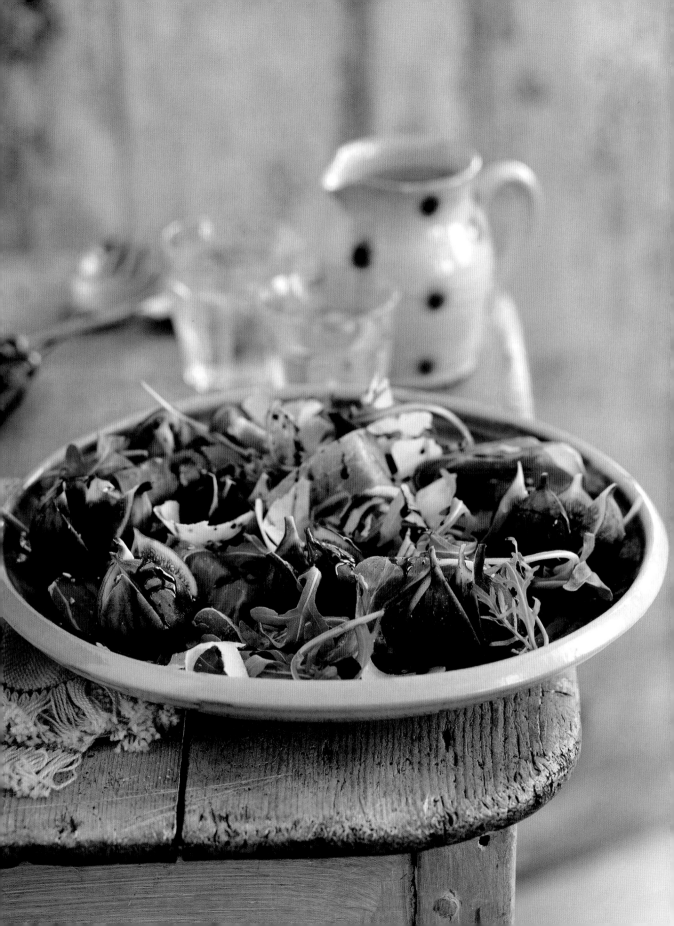

Mint and courgette frittata

SERVES 4

EASY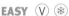

Syns per serving
Extra Easy: Free
Green: Free
Original: 2½ Syns

Preparation time: 15–20 minutes
Cooking time: under 25 minutes

2 medium potatoes, peeled and
cut into 1cm/½in dice
low calorie cooking spray
1 medium courgette, cut into
1cm/½in dice
6 large eggs
a small handful of mint,
roughly chopped
1 red chilli, deseeded and
roughly chopped
salt and freshly ground black pepper

The combination of eggs, mint and courgette is a marriage made in heaven.

Cook the potatoes in a pan of lightly salted boiling water for 6 minutes or until just cooked, then drain and set aside.

Spray a medium, deep, ovenproof frying pan with low calorie cooking spray and stir-fry the courgette for 4–5 minutes or until it is lightly browned. Add the potatoes and fry for 1–2 minutes.

In a bowl, beat the eggs, mint and red chilli together and season well.

Preheat the grill to medium-high.

Pour the egg mixture into the frying pan and stir briefly. Cook for 5 minutes over a low heat or until the bottom of the frittata has just started to set.

Transfer the pan to the grill and cook for 3–4 minutes or until golden and set.

Cut into wedges and serve warm or at room temperature.

Ham and red pepper frittata

SERVES 4

EASY ✳

Syns per serving
Extra Easy: Free
Original: Free
Green: 6½ Syns

Preparation time: 15 minutes
Cooking time: under 15 minutes

6 large eggs
salt and freshly ground black pepper
low calorie cooking spray
1 red onion, peeled and finely chopped
200g/7oz bottled roasted red peppers
in brine, drained
400g/14oz lean ham, roughly chopped
100g/3½oz quark
1 tsp paprika
a small handful of chopped mixed
herbs (chives, parsley and tarragon)
a crisp green salad, to serve

Easy to make and can be prepared in advance, this frittata is perfect food for a picnic, as it is extremely portable.

Beat the eggs in a mixing bowl and season well.

Spray a medium non-stick frying pan with low calorie cooking spray and place over a medium heat. Cook the onion for 3–4 minutes to soften, add the peppers, ham and eggs and cook for a further 5–6 minutes until almost set.

Preheat the grill to medium-high. Dot the quark on the top of the frittata, then scatter the paprika and herbs over the top and slide under the grill for 2–3 minutes until set and golden.

Cut into wedges and serve warm or at room temperature with a crisp green salad.

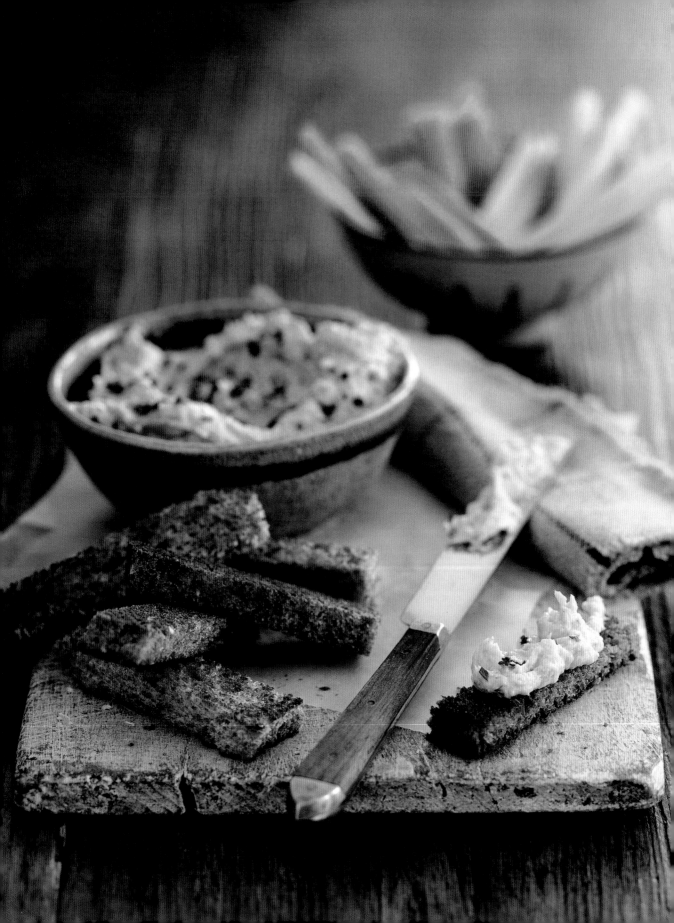

Salmon pâté with crudités

SERVES 4

EASY ✳

Syns per serving
Extra Easy: ½ Syn
Original: ½ Syn
Green: 9½ Syns

Preparation time: 10 minutes
Cooking time: under 20 minutes

400g/14oz salmon fillets, skinned
1 bay leaf
3 garlic cloves, peeled
1 tsp dried red chilli flakes
150g/5oz quark
4 level tbsp extra light mayonnaise
2 tbsp finely chopped flat-leaf parsley
juice of 1 lemon
wholemeal toast soldiers,
to serve (optional)

FOR THE CRUDITÉS
1 large carrot, peeled and
cut into batons
2 celery sticks, cut into batons

You can substitute cod fillets for the salmon if you want to ring a change in this recipe.

Place the salmon fillets in a saucepan with the bay leaf, garlic cloves and chilli flakes. Add enough cold water to cover and bring to the boil.

Reduce the heat to low and simmer gently for 15 minutes or until the salmon is cooked through. Drain the mixture through a fine sieve and transfer to a food processor. Add the quark, mayonnaise, parsley and lemon juice and process until fairly smooth.

Transfer the pâté to a serving bowl and serve with the vegetable crudités and wholemeal soldiers (3 Syns per 25g/1oz), if wished.

Chicken Milanese fingers with garlic mayonnaise

SERVES 4

EASY ❄

Syns per serving
Extra Easy: 3½ Syns
Original: 3½ Syns
Green: 11 Syns

Preparation time: 25 minutes
Cooking time: 20 minutes

4 skinless chicken breast fillets
low calorie cooking spray
4 slices wholemeal bread (from a
small 400g loaf)
4 tbsp finely chopped oregano
salt and freshly ground black pepper
2 large eggs, beaten
lemon wedges, to serve

FOR THE GARLIC MAYONNAISE
4 level tbsp extra light mayonnaise
100g/3½oz fat free natural
fromage frais
2 garlic cloves, peeled and crushed
juice of 1 lemon

This delicious chicken snack also makes a great mid-morning brunch or light lunch.

Preheat the oven to 200°C/Gas 6 and line a baking sheet with non-stick baking parchment.

Cut each chicken breast lengthways into 4 or 5 'fingers' and place in a bowl. Spray with low calorie cooking spray and stir to coat evenly.

Place the bread in a food processor and blend until finely crumbed. Transfer to a bowl, stir in the chopped oregano and season to taste.

Toss the chicken with the beaten eggs and turn to coat evenly. Arrange on the prepared baking sheet and sprinkle over the breadcrumb mixture and pat onto the chicken pieces. Spray with low calorie cooking spray.

Bake in the oven for 20 minutes, or until nicely browned and cooked through.

Meanwhile, make the garlic mayonnaise by mixing all the ingredients together in a bowl. Season well.

Serve the chicken fingers hot or at room temperature with the garlic mayonnaise and lemon wedges to squeeze over.

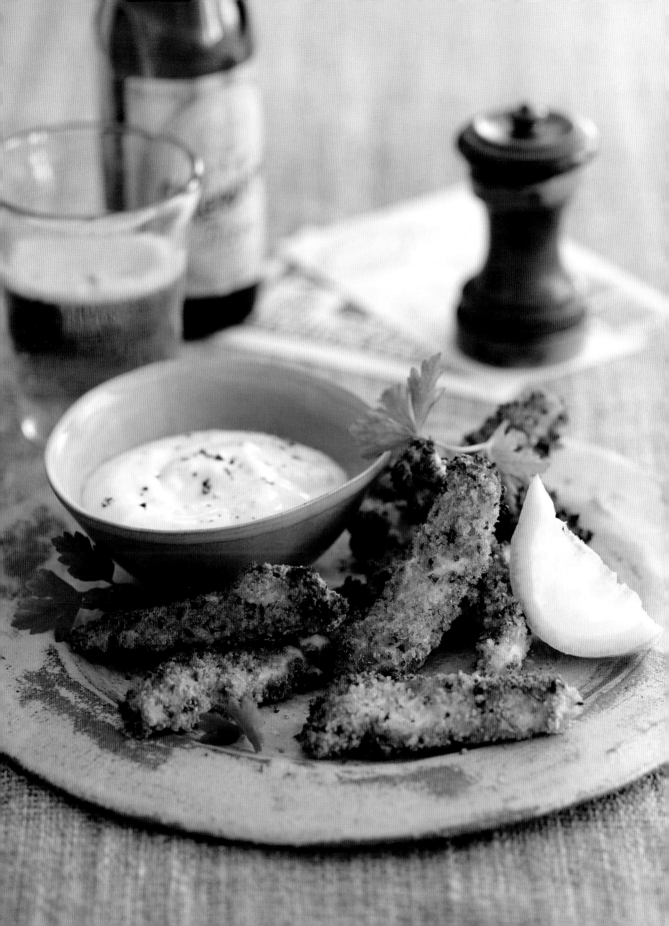

Chicken liver crostini

SERVES 4

EASY ❄

This tasty snack is the Tuscan version of chicken liver pâté and is delicious served on warm toasted bread.

Syns per serving
Extra Easy: 3 Syns
Original: 3 Syns
Green: 7 Syns

Preparation time: 15 minutes
Cooking time: 8–10 minutes

300g/11oz chicken livers
low calorie cooking spray
1 celery stick, finely chopped
1 shallot, peeled and finely chopped
2 garlic cloves, peeled and finely chopped
a pinch of nutmeg
2 tbsp very finely chopped flat-leaf parsley
100g/3½oz fat free natural fromage frais
salt and freshly ground black pepper
4 slices wholemeal bead (from a small 400g loaf)
wild rocket leaves, to garnish

Trim the chicken livers of any gristle, rinse and pat dry with kitchen paper.

Spray a large non-stick frying pan with low calorie cooking spray and place over a medium heat. Add the chicken livers, celery, shallot and garlic and stir-fry for 8–10 minutes.

Transfer this mixture to a food processor with the nutmeg, parsley and fromage frais. Process until fairly smooth, season well and then transfer to a bowl.

Make the crostini by toasting both sides of the bread (you can also do this on a hot griddle) and then cut each slice into two pieces.

Spread the chicken mixture over the crostini and serve immediately, garnished with rocket leaves.

Pork and herb loaf with tomato and basil salsa

You can make this rustic Tuscan-style snack using any lean minced meat of your choice instead of the pork, if desired.

SERVES 4–6

EASY ❆

Syns per serving (serves 4)
Extra Easy: Free
Original: Free
Green: 12 Syns

Syns per serving (serves 6)
Extra Easy: Free
Original: Free
Green: 8 Syns

Preparation time: 20 minutes
Cooking time: 1 hour

1 onion, peeled and finely chopped
2 garlic cloves, peeled and crushed
4 tbsp finely chopped flat-leaf parsley
2 tbsp finely chopped fresh oregano or
2 tsp dried oregano
500g/1lb 2oz extra lean minced pork
1 large egg, lightly beaten
8 rashers of lean back bacon, all
visible fat removed

FOR THE SALSA
4 ripe plum tomatoes, finely chopped
4 tbsp finely chopped basil
1 tbsp red wine vinegar
salt and freshly ground black pepper

Preheat the oven to 190°C/Gas 5.

Make the salsa by combining the tomatoes, basil and vinegar in a bowl. Season well, cover and stand at room temperature until needed.

Place the onion, garlic and herbs into the food processor and process until finely chopped. Transfer to a mixing bowl with the minced pork and egg. Finely chop 2 of the bacon rashers and add to the pork and season well. Mix well.

Use the rest of the bacon to line a 1.5 litre/ 2½ pint loaf tin, allowing the slices to hang over the sides. Spoon in the meatloaf mix and press down well. Fold the overhanging bacon over the top of the meatloaf and then put the loaf tin into a roasting tray.

Pour hot water into the roasting tray to come halfway up the side of the loaf tin and bake for 1 hour or until the loaf shrinks from the sides of tin.

Cool in the tin for 10 minutes, then drain off any excess liquid and turn out onto a board. Cut into thick slices and serve warm or cold with the salsa.

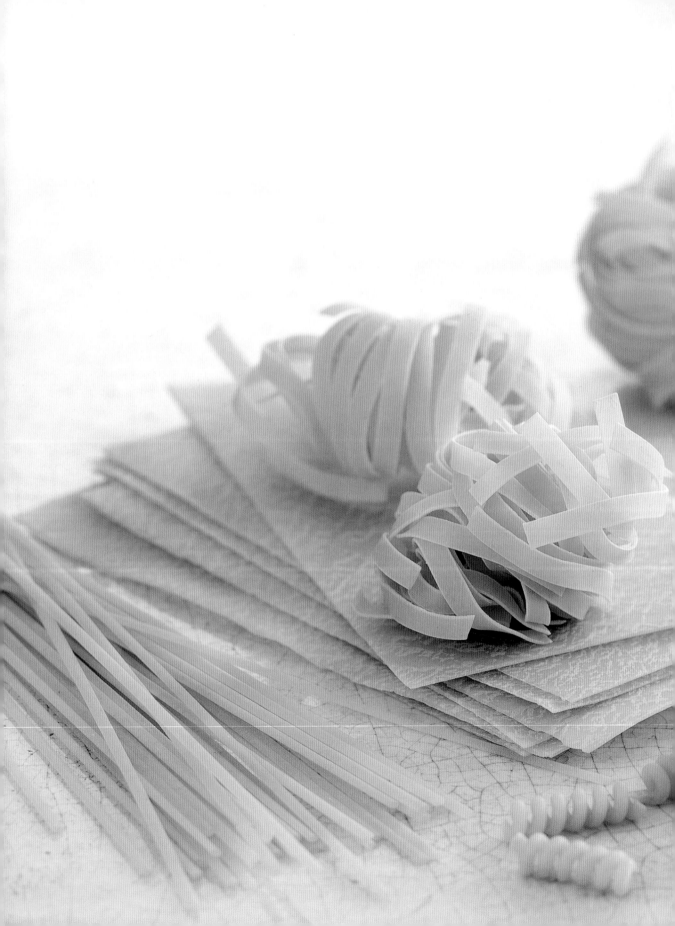

Chapter 3

Pasta and risottos

Everyone loves the classics such as spaghetti bolognese and lasagne, but pasta and risotto dishes have so much more to offer. Dishes such as Creamy Smoked Salmon Bucatini with Dill or Pumpkin, Chilli and Sage Risotto (see pages 86 and 102) are really special and just as easy to prepare as traditional favourites. Experiment with different types of pasta combinations, from Fusilli with Tuna, Capers and Mint to Italian-style Penne with Grilled Chicken Livers (see pages 90 and 91), or make delicious creamy risottos flavoured with wild mushrooms, ham or leek, or even red wine. And there's nothing like spicy sauces such as puttanesca or arrabiata to send your taste buds wild!

Quick pasta primavera

SERVES 4

EASY Ⓥ ⊛

Syns per serving
Extra Easy: Free
Green: Free
Original: 20½ Syns

Preparation time: 10 minutes
Cooking time: under 20 minutes

400g/14oz dried penne
low calorie cooking spray
1 garlic clove, peeled and crushed
200g/7oz asparagus, hard stalks
removed, blanched and cut
into bite-sized pieces
150g/5oz fresh peas, shelled
100g/3½oz frozen soya beans,
defrosted
100g/3½oz baby spinach leaves
finely grated zest and juice of 1 lemon
a large handful of spring herbs (basil,
dill, mint and parsley), chopped
salt and freshly ground black pepper

Packed with fresh spring vegetables and
full of flavour, this pasta dish is sure to
become a family favourite.

Cook the pasta according to the packet
instructions, drain, reserving 4–5 tablespoons
of the cooking liquid, and keep warm.

Spray a large non-stick frying pan with low calorie
cooking spray and place over a medium heat.
Add the garlic and fry for 1 minute.

Add the asparagus, peas, soya beans and spinach
and stir-fry for 1–2 minutes, until the spinach has
wilted slightly.

Add the drained pasta and the reserved cooking
liquid to the pan and stir to combine.

Stir in the lemon zest and juice and the chopped
herbs and season to taste.

Serve immediately.

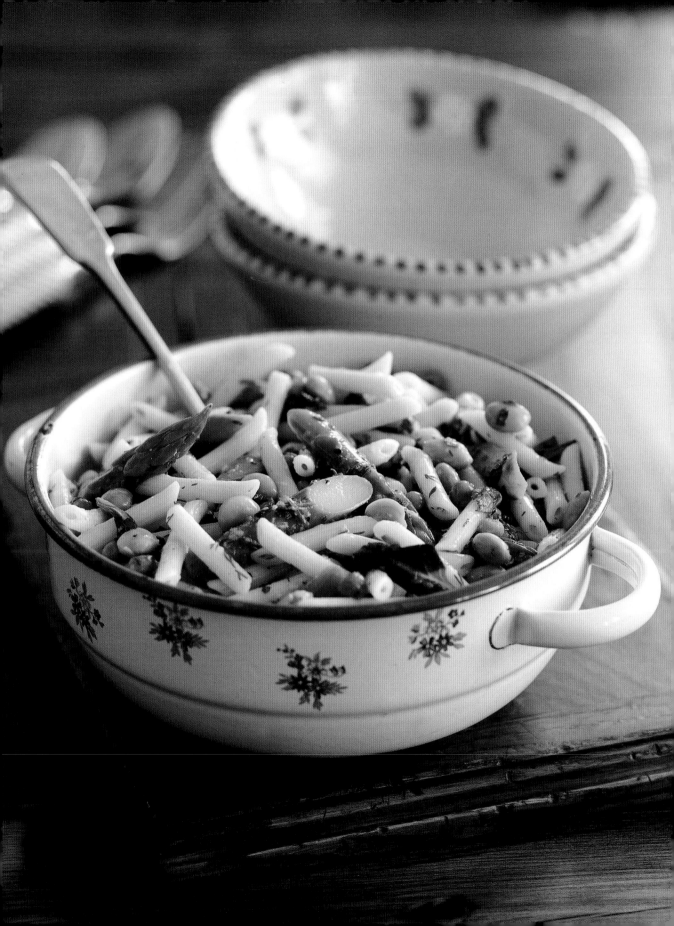

Penne al'arrabiata

SERVES 4

EASY Ⓥ ❋

Syns per serving
Extra Easy: Free
Green: Free
Original: 17 Syns

Preparation time: 10 minutes
Cooking time: under 25 minutes

2 medium hot red chillies, deseeded
and finely sliced
2 garlic cloves, peeled and chopped
600g/1lb 5oz canned
chopped tomatoes
a large handful of fresh basil
salt
400g/14oz dried penne
Parmesan shavings, to serve (optional)

Pasta is the ultimate fast food and this dish with tomatoes and chillies is ideal to cook after work when you're hungry and short of time. If you like your food hot, you can leave the seeds in the chillies.

Add the red chillies, garlic, tomatoes and basil to a large non-stick saucepan and place over a high heat.

Reduce the heat to medium and continue to cook, stirring often, for 20 minutes. Season to taste with salt.

Meanwhile, cook the pasta according to the packet instructions. Drain the pasta and stir into the tomato sauce.

Serve with Parmesan shavings (3 Syns per 15g/½oz), if desired.

Pasta puttanesca

SERVES 4

EASY ✳

Syns per serving
Extra Easy: ½ Syn
Green: 1 Syn
Original: 15 Syns

Preparation time: 15 minutes
Cooking time: under 20 minutes

low calorie cooking spray
2 red chillies, deseeded and
finely chopped
6 canned anchovy fillets in oil, drained
and chopped
2 garlic cloves, peeled and thinly sliced
500g/1lb 2oz ripe tomatoes, peeled,
deseeded and thickly sliced
8 black olives, pitted and sliced
2 tbsp capers, rinsed
350g/12oz dried spaghetti or linguine
2 tbsp finely chopped flat-leaf parsley
grated Parmesan cheese,
to serve (optional)

Famously named after 'ladies of the night', this robust dish is best matched by a glass of full-bodied, red wine.

Spray a large frying pan with low calorie cooking spray and place over a medium-low heat. Add the red chillies, anchovies and garlic. Gently stir-fry for 30 seconds, mashing the anchovies to a paste with a wooden spoon and taking care not to let the garlic brown.

Raise the heat to medium-high and add the tomatoes, olives and capers. Bring to the boil, then lower the heat and simmer for about 5 minutes.

Cook the pasta according to the packet instructions and drain well.

Pour the sauce into a serving dish, add the drained pasta and stir to combine.

Sprinkle with the parsley and grated Parmesan, (1½ Syns per level tbsp), if using, and serve immediately.

Pasta alla genovese

This classic pasta dish from Genoa combines the shaped trofie pasta with pesto, green beans, potatoes and vegetables of your choice.

SERVES 4

EASY ✳

Syns per serving
Extra Easy: 6 Syns
Green: 6 Syns
Original: 25½ Syns

Preparation time: 20 minutes
Cooking time: under 20 minutes

400g/14oz dried trofie pasta
2 medium potatoes, peeled and cut into 1cm/½in cubes
2–3 carrots, peeled and cut into 1cm/½in cubes
110g/4oz green beans, cut into 4cm/1½in lengths

FOR THE PESTO
75g/3oz basil
4 garlic cloves, peeled and crushed
110g/4oz Parmesan or Pecorino cheese, grated (or a mixture of the two)
2–3 garlic cloves
100ml/3½fl oz fat free vinaigrette
100ml/3½fl oz hot vegetable stock

First make the pesto by placing all the ingredients in a food processor and blending until fairly smooth. Transfer into a bowl and set aside.

To cook the pasta, bring a large pan of well-salted water to the boil, then add the pasta. Trofie pasta takes about 15 minutes to cook so, after 8–9 minutes, add the potatoes and carrots and bring back to the boil.

Allow to boil for 2 minutes, then add the green beans and cook for another 3–4 minutes.

By the time the trofie is cooked but still firm the vegetables will be nicely cooked. Drain thoroughly and toss the pasta together with the pesto.

Serve with extra grated Parmesan (1½ Syns per level tbsp) or Pecorino cheese (2 Syns per level tbsp) and a sprig of fresh basil, if desired.

Tip If you can't find trofie pasta, use any short-shaped pasta instead.

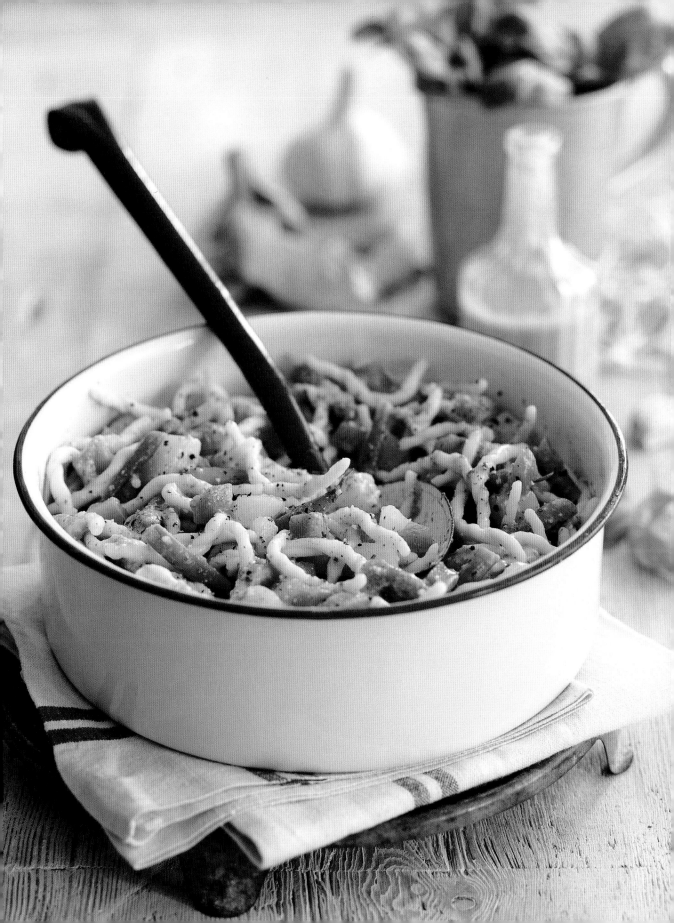

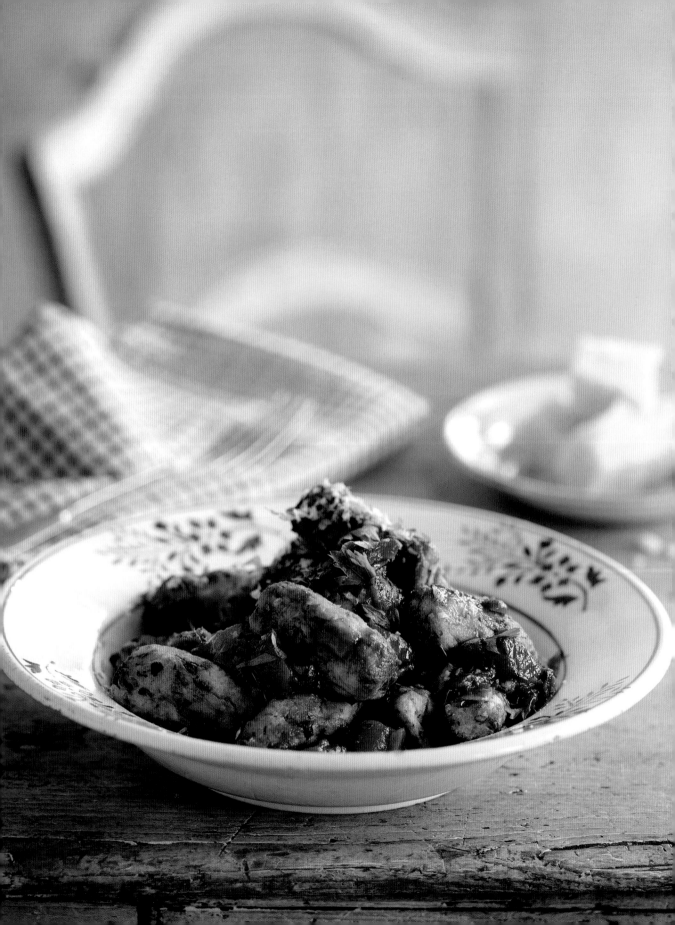

Potato gnocchi with red pepper sauce

SERVES 4

WORTH THE EFFORT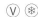

Syns per serving
Extra Easy: Free
Green: Free
Original: 9½ Syns

Preparation time: about 1 hour plus overnight chilling
Cooking time: under 30 minutes

FOR THE GNOCCHI
1kg/2lb 4oz Desiree potatoes
1 tsp dried oregano
8 tbsp finely chopped parsley
2 spring onions, trimmed and very finely sliced
1 large egg, lightly beaten
salt and freshly ground black pepper
low calorie cooking spray
finely chopped flat-leaf parsley
grated Parmesan cheese (optional)

FOR THE RED PEPPER SAUCE
400g/14oz bottled roasted red pepper in brine, rinsed, drained and roughly chopped
300g/11oz passata with garlic and herbs
1 onion, peeled and finely diced
3 garlic cloves, peeled and crushed
1 tsp crushed dried red chilli flakes
6 tbsp finely chopped basil

These baked potato dumplings are flavoured with herbs and spring onion and simply served with a piquant red pepper sauce.

Place the potatoes in a large saucepan, cover with water and bring to the boil. Cook for 25–35 minutes or until the potatoes are tender.

Drain and, when cool, peel off the skins and place the potatoes in a large wide bowl. Mash until fairly smooth. Add the dried oregano, parsley, spring onions and egg. Season well and mash until well combined. Cover and chill in the fridge overnight.

Make the red pepper sauce by placing all the sauce ingredients in a heavy-based saucepan. Bring to the boil and cook over a high heat for 15–20 minutes, stirring often. Season well and remove from the heat and keep warm.

When ready to cook the gnocchi, preheat the oven to 200°C/Gas 6 and line a baking tray with non-stick baking parchment.

Make the gnocchi by taking small walnut-sized pieces from the mixture and shaping them into balls or cylindrical shapes. Place them in a single layer on the baking tray, spray lightly with low calorie cooking spray and bake in the oven for 10–12 minutes or until lightly browned.

Serve the gnocchi with the sauce spooned over. Sprinkle over the parsley and Parmesan cheese (1½ Syns per level tbsp), if using.

Creamy smoked salmon bucatini with dill

SERVES 4

EASY ✳

Syns per serving
Extra Easy: Free
Green: 2½ Syns
Original: 14½ Syns

Preparation time: 20 minutes
Cooking time: under 20 minutes

low calorie cooking spray
6 spring onions, trimmed and finely chopped
150ml/5fl oz vegetable stock
200g/7oz quark
salt and freshly ground black pepper
2 garlic cloves, peeled and crushed
a pinch of nutmeg
4 tbsp finely chopped dill
juice of ½ lemon
500g/1lb 2oz runner beans, trimmed and thinly sliced
350g/12oz dried bucatini or spirali pasta
150g/5oz smoked salmon, cut into small strips (or use smoked salmon trimmings)

This pretty and tasty pasta dish can be made using any smoked fish of your choice, but smoked salmon adds a delicate flavour.

Spray a large non-stick frying pan with low calorie cooking spray, then fry the spring onions for 1 minute, until softened. Add the stock and boil hard for 2–3 minutes.

Stir in the quark, season well and add the garlic and nutmeg. Bring to the boil and simmer for 2–3 minutes until slightly thickened. Stir in the dill and lemon juice. Set aside.

Blanch the runner beans in lightly salted boiling water for 4–5 minutes. Drain and refresh under cold running water.

Cook the pasta according to the packet instructions. Drain well, reserving a little of the cooking liquid.

Toss the hot pasta with the drained runner beans, smoked salmon and the dill sauce, loosening with a couple of spoonfuls of the pasta's cooking liquid, if necessary. The heat of the pasta should reheat the sauce and slightly cook the smoked salmon, but stir over a gentle heat to warm through, if necessary. Serve immediately.

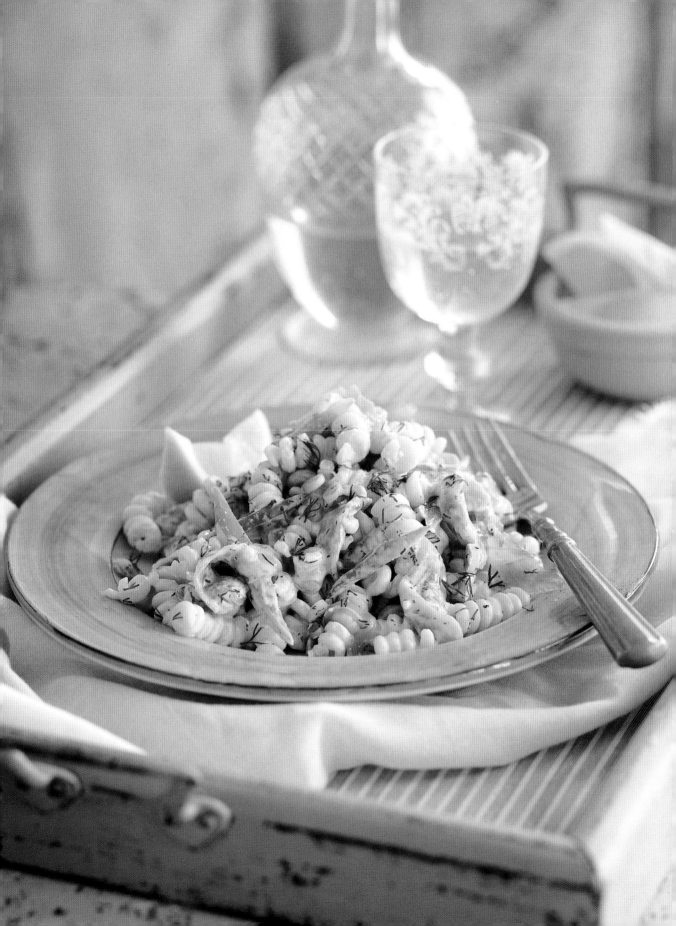

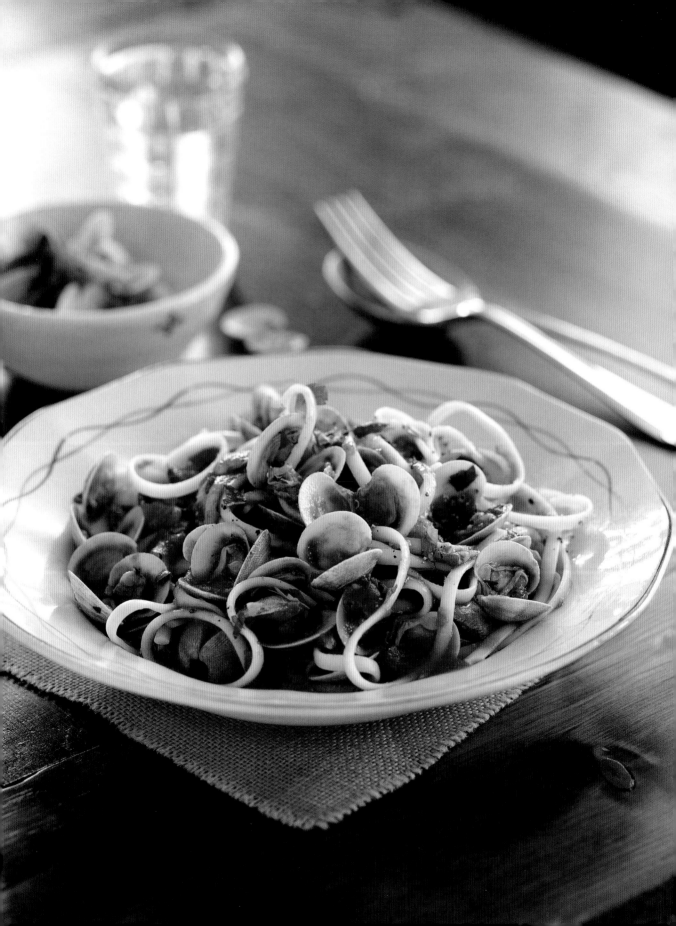

Linguine vongole

SERVES 4

EASY

Syns per serving
Extra Easy: Free
Green: 3½ Syns
Original: 17 Syns

Preparation time: 20 minutes
Cooking time: under 40 minutes

40 very small fresh clams
low calorie cooking spray
2 garlic cloves, peeled and
finely chopped
1 level tsp anchovy paste
2 tbsp finely chopped parsley
400g can chopped tomatoes
400g/14oz dried linguine
chopped parsley, to serve

Long pasta is the choice for seafood dishes around coastal Italy. This simple yet delicious dish is made with fresh clams, but you could use mussels instead for variety.

Scrub the clams, discarding any that remain open when tapped sharply. Place them in a pan over a high heat. Add 100ml/3½fl oz of water, cover with a lid and cook for 3–4 minutes, shaking the pan occasionally, or until all the shells have opened. Discard any clams that have not opened after 5 minutes.

Strain the clam juices from the pan through a sieve lined with muslin or kitchen paper and reserve the liquid.

Spray a large non-stick saucepan with low calorie cooking spray and place over a medium heat. Add the garlic and stir-fry for 1 minute or until the garlic begins to colour, then add the anchovy paste and chopped parsley and stir-fry for about 30 seconds.

Add the tomatoes and the strained clam juices. Bring to the boil, then reduce the heat and simmer for 20–25 minutes.

Cook the linguine according to the packet instructions and drain well.

Add the clam flesh to the tomato sauce and stir well. Then stir the sauce into the cooked pasta and serve immediately sprinkled with chopped parsley.

Fusilli with tuna, capers and mint

SERVES 4

EASY ✽

Syns per serving (without anchovies)
Extra Easy: Free
Green: 5½ Syns
Original: 17 Syns

Syns per serving (with anchovies)
Extra Easy: Free
Green: 6 Syns
Original: 17 Syns

Preparation time: 15 minutes
Cooking time: under 20 minutes

low calorie cooking spray
1 dried chilli, deseeded and crumbled
2 tsp of dried oregano
2 garlic cloves, peeled and chopped
6 canned anchovy fillets in oil, drained and chopped (optional)
400g can cherry tomatoes
400g can tuna in spring water, drained
2 tbsp capers, rinsed
salt and freshly ground black pepper
400g/14oz dried fusilli
2 tbsp finely chopped mint

This tasty and quick to cook pasta dish is made mostly from store cupboard ingredients.

Spray a non-stick frying pan with low calorie cooking spray and sauté the chilli, oregano and garlic for 1 minute.

Add the anchovy fillets, if using, and, over a low heat, mash the ingredients together against the side of the pan with a spoon. Cook for a further 2 minutes.

Stir in the cherry tomatoes and cook for another 2–3 minutes before mixing in the tuna and capers. Heat for a further 5 minutes, stirring frequently, and season well.

Meanwhile, cook the pasta according to the packet instructions and drain.

Transfer the pasta to a serving dish and spoon over the sauce. Serve scattered with the mint.

Italian-style penne with grilled chicken livers

In this recipe, spiced grilled chicken livers are tossed with fresh tomatoes and basil and served over freshly cooked penne.

SERVES 4

EASY ❄

Syns per serving
Extra Easy: Free
Green: 5 Syns
Original: 14½ Syns

Preparation time: 15 minutes plus marinating
Cooking time: under 20 minutes

400g/14oz chicken livers, trimmed and cut into 2cm/¾in dice
3 tsp paprika
2 tsp ground cumin
1 tsp ground cinnamon
1 tsp dried oregano
juice of 1 lemon
salt and freshly ground black pepper
2 ripe tomatoes, finely chopped
a small handful of roughly chopped basil
low calorie cooking spray
350g/12oz dried penne

Place the chicken livers in a large ceramic bowl and add the paprika, cumin, cinnamon, oregano and lemon juice. Season well and toss to combine. Cover and marinate for 1 hour.

Place the tomatoes in a separate large bowl with the basil.

Preheat the grill to medium-high. Line a grill rack with foil and spread the chicken liver mixture over it in a single layer. Spray with low calorie cooking spray and cook under the grill for 2–3 minutes on each side or until just cooked through.

Remove from the grill, add to the tomato and basil mixture with any juices, cover with foil and keep warm.

Meanwhile, cook the pasta according to the packet instructions. Drain well, toss with the chicken liver mixture and serve immediately.

Chunky oven-baked ragu tagliatelle

SERVES 4

EASY ❄

Syns per serving
Extra Easy: Free
Green: 10½ Syns
Original: 17 Syns

Preparation time: 15 minutes
Cooking time: just over 2 hours

low calorie cooking spray
250g/9oz extra lean minced beef
250g/9oz extra lean minced pork
200g/7oz chicken livers, trimmed and
roughly chopped
400g can chopped tomatoes
1 large carrot, peeled and
roughly diced
2 celery sticks, roughly chopped
1 onion, peeled and roughly chopped
2 tsp dried thyme
2 tsp dried oregano
salt and freshly ground black pepper
400g/14oz dried tagliatelle

This is a typical Italian peasants' dish from southern Italy with robust flavours, colours and textures. When fresh plum tomatoes are in season, use them instead of canned ones for a wonderful, fresh flavour.

Preheat the oven to 150°C/Gas 2. Spray a large non-stick frying pan with low calorie cooking spray and place over a high heat. Stir-fry the minced beef until browned and transfer to a deep ovenproof dish.

Add the minced pork to the frying pan and cook until browned then add to the beef in the ovenproof dish.

Add the liver to the pan and cook until browned then add to the beef and pork.

Mix together the tomatoes, carrot, celery, onion and dried herbs, season well and stir into the meat mixture. Cover, place in the oven and cook for 2 hours, stirring every 20–30 minutes.

When almost ready to serve, cook the tagliatelle according to the packet instructions, drain and serve immediately with the chunky sauce spooned over.

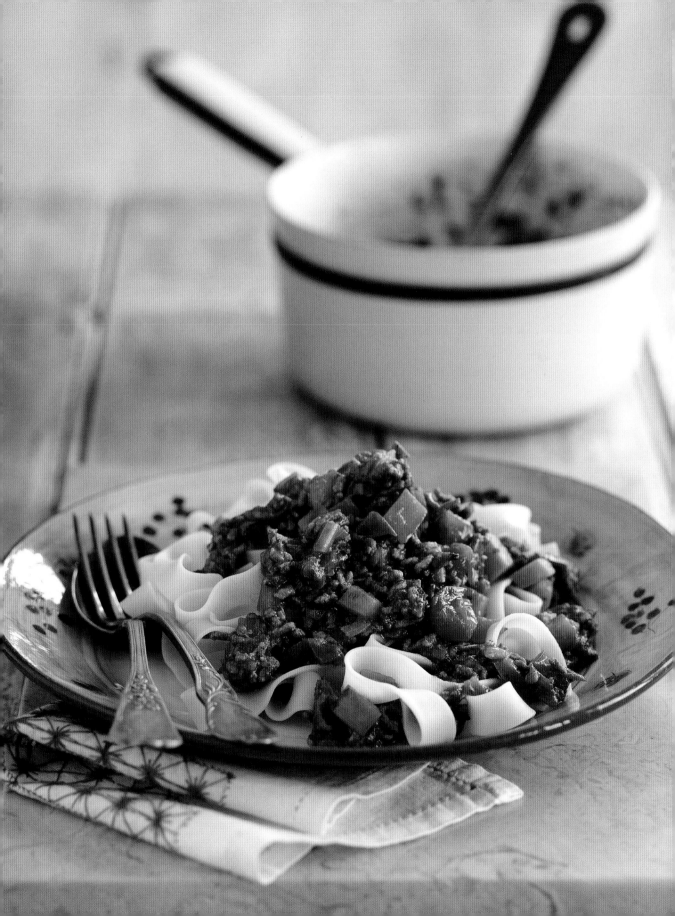

Prosciutto pappardelle

SERVES 4

EASY ✳

Syns per serving
Extra Easy: 1 Syn
Green: 2½ Syns
Original: 15½ Syns

Preparation time: 10 minutes
Cooking time: under 20 minutes

350g/12oz dried pappardelle
low calorie cooking spray
6 slices lean prosciutto, cut crosswise
into 1cm/½in wide strips
16 cos lettuce leaves, cut across into
3cm/1¼in wide strips
2 cloves garlic, peeled and finely sliced
150ml/5fl oz chicken stock
3 spring onions, trimmed and
finely sliced
300g/11oz green beans, trimmed and
cut into 2cm/¾in lengths
2 tbsp freshly chopped flat-leaf parsley
salt and freshly ground black pepper
grated Parmesan cheese,
to serve (optional)

In this unusual but delicious summer pasta dish, prosciutto, lettuce and green beans are tossed with stock and served with pappardelle.

Cook the pasta according to the packet instructions. Drain and keep warm.

Meanwhile, spray a wide non-stick frying pan with low calorie cooking spray. Add the prosciutto and gently stir-fry for 4–5 minutes.

Add the lettuce and garlic, cover the pan and cook gently for about 3 minutes until the lettuce has wilted.

Add the stock, spring onions and green beans, bring to the boil and cook gently for 5 minutes or until the spring onions and green beans are just tender.

Toss in the drained pasta and chopped parsley and season well. Toss to combine and tip into a serving dish.

Serve immediately with grated Parmesan (1½ Syns per level tbsp), if desired.

Spaghetti alla carbonara

In this classic recipe, the heat from the pasta effectively cooks the egg as you toss the hot spaghetti with the creamy, bacon-flecked sauce.

SERVES 4

EASY

Syns per serving
Extra Easy: 5½ Syns
Green: 8½ Syns
Original: 22½ Syns

Preparation time: 10 minutes
Cooking time: under 10 minutes

salt
400g/14oz dried spaghetti
low calorie cooking spray
175g/6oz rashers of lean bacon, all visible fat removed and cut into 5mm/¼in strips
3 garlic cloves, peeled and finely chopped
a small handful of flat-leaf parsley, finely chopped
3 large eggs, lightly beaten
110g/4oz Pecorino cheese, finely grated
freshly ground black pepper

Bring a large saucepan of lightly salted water to the boil. Add the spaghetti and cook according to the packet instructions.

Spray a large, deep frying pan with low calorie cooking spray and place over a medium-high heat. Add the bacon strips and fry until they are lightly golden.

Add the garlic and parsley and cook for a few seconds. Remove from the heat and set aside.

Drain the spaghetti well, tip into the frying pan with the bacon, garlic and parsley, add the beaten eggs and half of the grated cheese and toss together well.

Season to taste with a little salt and black pepper. The heat from the spaghetti will be sufficient to partly cook the egg, but still leave it moist and creamy. Take to the table and serve sprinkled with the rest of the cheese.

Rigatoni with rich oxtail stew

SERVES 4

EASY ✲

Syns per serving
Extra Easy: Free
Green: 11½ Syns
Original: 14½ Syns

Preparation time: 20 minutes
Cooking time: just over 3 hours

low calorie cooking spray
2 oxtails (about 2kg/4lb 8oz), jointed,
trimmed of all visible fat and
cut into pieces
2 onions, peeled and finely chopped
3 carrots, peeled and roughly chopped
3 celery sticks, roughly chopped
2 garlic cloves, peeled and
finely chopped
400g can chopped tomatoes
200ml/7fl oz beef stock
2 bay leaves
2 thyme sprigs
salt and freshly ground black pepper
350g/12oz dried rigatoni

Long, slow cooking makes for a meltingly rich and tender oxtail stew for the robust rigatoni pasta, which is one of the more popular dishes from Tuscany.

Preheat the oven to 180°C/Gas 4.

Spray a large flameproof casserole dish with low calorie cooking spray and, working in batches, brown the oxtail really well on all sides.

Remove from the pan with a slotted spoon and set aside. Add the onions, carrots, celery and garlic and fry for 3–4 minutes or until starting to colour.

Stir in the tomatoes, stock and herbs. Tip the meat back into the pan and season well. Cover the pan and braise in the oven for 3 hours or until the meat is meltingly tender.

About 10 minutes before the end of the oxtail cooking time, cook the rigatoni according to the packet instructions. Drain and serve with the rich oxtail stew spooned over.

Risi e bisi

SERVES 4

EASY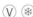

Syns per serving (without Parmesan)
Extra Easy: Free
Green: Free
Original: 13½ Syns

Syns per serving (with Parmesan)
Extra Easy: 6 Syns
Green: 6 Syns
Original: 19½ Syns

Preparation time: 15 minutes
Cooking time: under 30 minutes

1 small onion, peeled and
finely chopped
2 carrots, peeled and finely diced
1 celery stick, finely diced
2 garlic cloves, peeled and
finely chopped
1.5 litres/2½ pints boiling hot
vegetable stock
225g/8oz dried risotto rice
300g/11oz fresh or frozen peas
a small handful of
fresh parsley, chopped
110g/4oz Parmesan cheese,
grated (optional)
salt and freshly ground black pepper

This tasty and flavoursome dish of rice and peas is packed with colour, flavour and texture and is slightly 'wetter' than a normal risotto.

Place the onion, carrots, celery and garlic in a heavy-based saucepan and place over a high heat.

Add the stock and the rice, bring to the boil and simmer very gently for 15–20 minutes, stirring once or twice.

Stir in the peas and cook for a further 5 minutes or until the peas are tender.

Finally stir in the parsley and grated Parmesan, if using, and season well.

Ladle into soup bowls and eat immediately.

Red wine risotto

SERVES 4

EASY ❄

Syns per serving
Extra Easy: 7 Syns
Green: 7 Syns
Original: 18½ Syns

Preparation time: 5 minutes
Cooking time: under 30 minutes

low calorie cooking spray
1 onion, peeled and finely chopped
250g/9oz dried risotto rice
150ml/5fl oz Italian red wine
1 litre/1¾ pints vegetable stock
110g/4oz Parmesan cheese,
finely grated
salt and freshly ground black pepper
2 tbsp chopped parsley
a crisp green salad, to serve (optional)

This is an amazing risotto to serve on its own. Use good quality red wine for this dish – a full-bodied Italian Barolo or Chianti is perfect.

Spray a large saucepan with low calorie cooking spray and place over a medium heat. Add the onion and stir-fry fry gently for 4–5 minutes, until the onions are softened but not coloured.

Add the rice and stir for 1–2 minutes, then pour in the wine. Bring the mixture to the boil, then reduce the heat and simmer for 2–3 minutes, or until the wine has been absorbed by the rice.

Meanwhile, heat the stock in a separate saucepan until boiling, then reduce the heat and maintain the stock on a gentle simmer.

Add a ladleful of stock to the rice and bring to a simmer. Stir regularly until all of the stock has been absorbed. Repeat this process until all the stock has been used up and the rice is tender and the risotto is creamy. This should take 20–25 minutes.

Stir in the Parmesan cheese, reserving a little for garnish, and season to taste.

Sprinkle over the parsley and remaining Parmesan cheese and serve with the green salad, if wished.

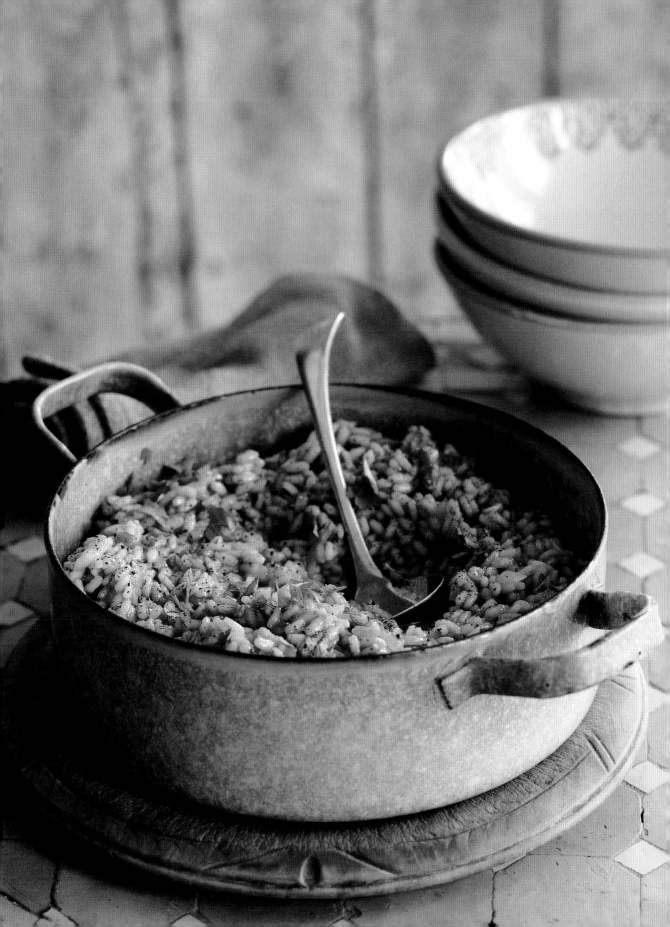

Baked spinach risotto

SERVES 4

EASY ✳

Syns per serving
Extra Easy: 6 Syns
Green: 6 Syns
Original: 20 Syns

Preparation time: 10 minutes
Cooking time: 30–35 minutes

low calorie cooking spray
8 spring onions, trimmed and
finely sliced
2 garlic cloves, peeled and
finely chopped
100g/3½oz spinach leaves,
finely chopped
300g/11oz dried risotto rice
3 tbsp dried Italian mixed herbs
salt and freshly ground black pepper
800ml/28fl oz boiling hot
vegetable stock
200g/7oz cherry tomatoes, halved
110g/4oz Parmesan cheese, grated

Leave this simple spinach and cherry tomato risotto to cook in the oven while you get on with something else – the result will be a wonderfully creamy risotto for very little effort.

Preheat the oven to 180°C/Gas 4.

Spray a large non-stick frying pan with low calorie cooking spray and place over a high heat. Stir in the onions, garlic and spinach and stir-fry for 6–7 minutes or until the spinach is almost wilted.

Add the rice and dried herbs and mix well until the rice is coated and season well.

Add the cherry tomatoes and the hot stock and give the pan a quick stir.

Transfer to an ovenproof dish, cover tightly with a lid and bake for 20–25 minutes or until the rice is cooked.

Stir in the Parmesan cheese and serve immediately.

Wild mushroom risotto

Any fresh wild mushrooms that are packed with flavour will taste wonderful in this risotto from Tuscany. However, it works equally well with reconstituted dried porcini mushrooms.

SERVES 4

EASY Ⓥ ❄

Syns per serving
Extra Easy: Free
Green: Free
Original: 10 Syns

Preparation time: 15 minutes
Cooking time: under 30 minutes

low calorie cooking spray
6 shallots, peeled and finely chopped
4 garlic cloves, peeled and finely chopped
225g/8oz dried risotto rice
400g/14oz mixed wild mushrooms, cut into bite-sized pieces
1.25 litres/2 pints boiling hot vegetable stock
salt and freshly ground black pepper
4 tbsp chopped flat-leaf parsley
1 tbsp chopped tarragon

Spray a large non-stick frying pan with low calorie cooking spray and place over a medium heat. Add the shallots and garlic and stir-fry for 3–4 minutes.

Add the rice and mushrooms and stir-fry for 2–3 minutes. Add a large ladleful of the stock and stir and cook until the liquid is absorbed. Repeat adding a ladleful at a time until all the stock is used up and the rice is creamy and tender but still retaining a bite. This should take about 20–25 minutes.

Remove from the heat, season well and stir in the chopped herbs and serve in warmed bowls.

Pumpkin, chilli and sage risotto

SERVES 4

EASY ⓥ ⊛

Syns per serving
Extra Easy: Free
Green: Free
Original: 11½ Syns

Preparation time: 15 minutes
Cooking time: about 30 minutes

low calorie cooking spray
1 onion, peeled and finely diced
1 carrot, peeled and finely diced
1 celery stick, finely diced
2 garlic cloves, peeled and thinly sliced
300g/11oz pumpkin flesh,
cut into 2cm/¾in dice
1 red chilli, deseeded and
finely chopped
250g/9oz dried risotto rice
1.25 litres/2 pints vegetable stock
2 tbsp finely chopped sage
salt and freshly ground black pepper
a crisp green salad, to serve (optional)

The simplicity of this dish appeals to most people and accounts for its popularity with children as well as grown-ups.

Spray a large saucepan with low calorie cooking spray and place over a medium heat. Add the onion, carrot, celery, garlic, pumpkin and red chilli and stir-fry gently for 4–5 minutes, until the vegetables are slightly softened but not coloured. Add the rice and stir for 1–2 minutes.

Meanwhile, heat the stock in a separate saucepan until boiling, then reduce the heat and maintain the stock on a gentle simmer.

Add a ladleful of stock to the rice along with the chopped sage and bring to a simmer. Stir regularly until all of the stock has been absorbed. Repeat this process until all of the stock has been used up and the rice is tender and the risotto is creamy. This should take 20–25 minutes.

Season to taste and serve with a crisp green salad, if wished.

Tip If pumpkin isn't available, this risotto works equally well with any type of squash. It is delicious served with grated Parmesan cheese (1½ Syns per level tbsp).

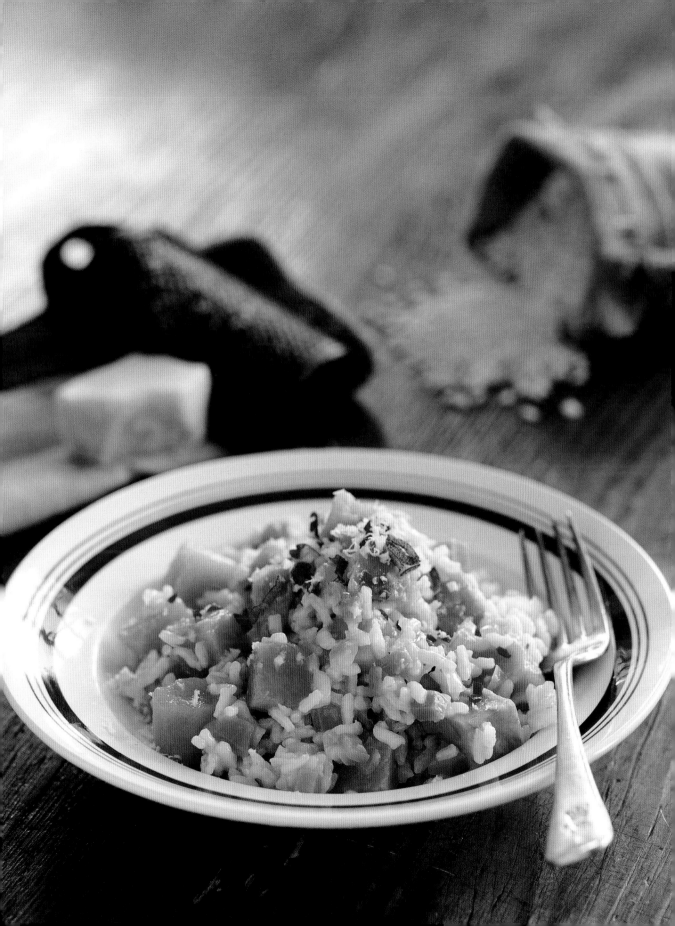

Seafood risotto

SERVES 4

EASY

Syns per serving
Extra Easy: Free
Green: 6½ Syns
Original: 10 Syns

Preparation time: 15 minutes
Cooking time: under 30 minutes

1 onion, peeled and finely chopped
2 garlic cloves, peeled and
finely chopped
1 fennel bulb, trimmed and
finely chopped
225g/8oz dried risotto rice
1.25 litres/2 pints boiling hot fish stock
2 x 300g packs frozen mixed seafood
(thawed) or 600g/1lb 5oz fresh mixed
seafood
6 spring onions, trimmed and
finely chopped
salt and freshly ground black pepper

Coastal Italy is home to great seafood risottos of many different kinds. This one from Liguria is simply flavoured with fennel, garlic and onion.

Place the onion, garlic and fennel in a wide, heavy-based saucepan and then add the rice. Place over a high heat and stir to mix well.

Add the hot stock to the rice and vegetables a ladleful at a time, stirring each time to give the risotto a creamy effect.

When the rice is almost cooked (about 20–25 minutes), add the seafood and spring onions. Stir and cook for 4–5 minutes, season well and remove from the heat.

Serve immediately ladled into warmed bowls.

Ham and leek risotto

SERVES 4

EASY ❋

Syns per serving
Extra Easy: Free
Green: 2 Syns
Original: 11½ Syns

Preparation time: 10 minutes
Cooking time: under 30 minutes

low calorie cooking spray
2 shallots, peeled and finely chopped
6 baby leeks, trimmed and finely sliced
1 carrot, peeled and finely diced
1 celery stick, finely diced
250g/9oz dried risotto rice
110g/4oz premium sliced lean ham,
roughly chopped
1.25 litres/2 pints chicken stock
salt and freshly ground black pepper
4 tbsp finely chopped chives

The delicate, sweet onion flavour of the leek complements the salty ham in this simple, yet delicious risotto.

Spray a large saucepan with low calorie cooking spray and place over a medium heat. Add the shallots, leeks, carrot and celery, and stir-fry gently for 4–5 minutes, until the vegetables are softened but not coloured. Add the rice and stir for 1–2 minutes, then add the ham.

Meanwhile, heat the stock in a separate saucepan until boiling, then reduce the heat and maintain the stock on a gentle simmer.

Add a ladleful of stock to the rice and bring to a simmer. Stir regularly until all the stock has been absorbed. Repeat this process until all the stock has been used up and the rice is tender and the risotto creamy. This should take 20–25 minutes.

Season to taste and sprinkle over the chives before serving.

Chapter 4

Fish and shellfish

Typical Italian fish and seafood dishes are simple to cook and full of robust flavours, as in Roasted Sea Bass with Basil and Roasted Vine Tomatoes or Griddled Squid Salad with Mint and Coriander (see pages 114 and 127). Oily fish like mackerel, fresh tuna and sardines are also popular, and are often grilled, roasted, baked or even served 'al cartoccio' (in a paper parcel), rather than fried, which makes them even healthier. Our recipes feature delicious ways to enjoy them, such as Baked Italian-style Sardines Beccafico, Ligurian Fish Stew, a rich tomato- and onion-based dish from the northwest of Italy, and Tuna al Cartoccio (see pages 109, 113 and 115).

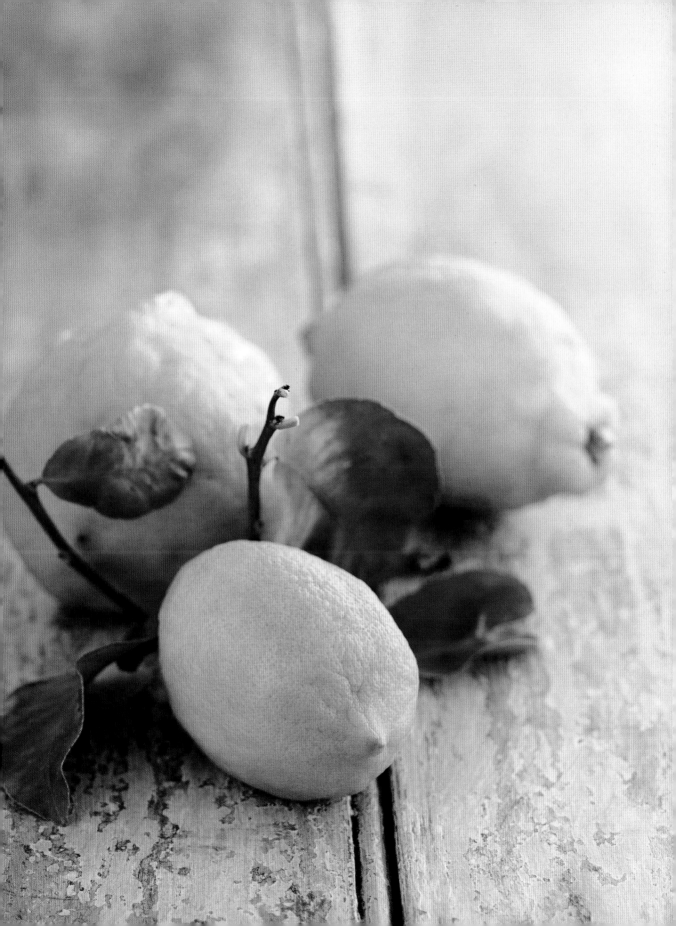

Baked coley with tomato, lemon and capers

SERVES 4

EASY ✳ (if fish not previously frozen)

Syns per serving
Extra Easy: Free
Original: Free
Green: 3½ Syns

Preparation time: 15 minutes
Cooking time: under 20 minutes

2 large coley fillets, skinned
salt and freshly ground black pepper
100ml/3½fl oz vegetable stock
1 lemon, peeled and segmented
2 plum tomatoes, finely chopped
2 tbsp capers, rinsed
2 tbsp finely chopped parsley
1 shallot, peeled and finely chopped
2 large hard-boiled eggs, finely chopped
a green salad, to serve

Firm-textured coley is ideal for grilling or barbecuing. Here it is served with a fresh, zesty sauce that complements its flavour.

Preheat the grill to medium-high. Season the coley fillets and place on a grill rack. Place under the grill and cook for 6–8 minutes or until the fish is cooked through. Remove to a serving platter, cover and keep warm.

Meanwhile, put the stock in a small saucepan and simmer until the liquid volume has reduced by half. Stir in the lemon segments, tomatoes, capers, parsley and shallot and season well.

Spoon the sauce over the fish and sprinkle over the chopped egg. Serve with the green salad.

Baked Italian-style sardines beccafico

SERVES 4

WORTH THE EFFORT ❄

Syns per serving
Extra Easy: 1 Syn
Original: 1 Syn
Green: 24½ Syns

Preparation time: 25 minutes plus marinating
Cooking time: under 20 minutes

8 medium-sized sardines, scaled, gutted and butterflied
low calorie cooking spray
mixed salad, to serve

FOR THE MARINADE
1 red chilli, deseeded and finely diced
juice of 2 oranges
juice of 1 lemon

FOR THE FILLING
2 garlic cloves, peeled and chopped
4 tbsp finely chopped flat-leaf parsley
4 tbsp finely chopped fennel bulb
2 tbsp finely chopped mint
2 tbsp small capers, rinsed
salt and freshly ground black pepper

FOR THE TOPPING
8 bay leaves
8 lemon slices
juice of 2 oranges
juice of 2 lemons

When opened up and boned, sardines cook in minutes in a hot oven. This is a good dish to prepare a day ahead, then cook and serve with a crisp green salad.

Preheat the oven to 180°C/Gas 4. Make the marinade by mixing all the ingredients together. Lay the sardines in a shallow dish and pour over the marinade. Leave for about 30 minutes in the fridge. Make the filling by mixing together all the ingredients in a bowl. Season to taste.

Remove the fish from the marinade and dry with kitchen paper. Lay them out, skin side down, season and sprinkle the filling over the fish.

Carefully roll up the fish and ensure you leave the tails sticking up in the air. Place a bay leaf and a slice of lemon on each, securing with a skewer or a cocktail stick.

Line an ovenproof dish with baking parchment and lay the fish on top. Spray with low calorie cooking spray and bake for 15–20 minutes or until the fish is just cooked through. Remove from the oven and pour over the orange and lemon juices. Serve immediately with a mixed salad.

Tip To butterfly the sardines, first remove the heads. Then lay out the fish, cut side down, and press down along the backbone with your thumb to loosen the bone. Turn the fish over and gently pull away the backbone, cutting it off at the tail. Remove any remaining small bones with tweezers, if desired.

Baked swordfish siciliana

Fish steaks benefit from being marinated before cooking, especially if you're baking them. You can substitute tuna in this recipe quite successfully if you want to ring a change.

SERVES 4

EASY ❄ (if fish not previously frozen)

Syns per serving
Extra Easy: 3½ Syns
Original: 3½ Syns
Green: 13 Syns

Preparation time: 20 minutes plus chilling
Cooking time: 10–12 minutes

4 x 175g/6oz swordfish steaks
finely grated zest and juice of 1 lemon
1 tsp dried red chilli flakes
2 tsp finely chopped mint
2 garlic cloves, peeled and crushed
sea salt

FOR THE SALSA
1 red chilli, deseeded and finely chopped
1 avocado, cut into 5mm/¼in dice
2 garlic cloves, peeled and finely chopped
1 small red onion, peeled, halved and thinly sliced
½ cucumber, cut into 5mm/¼in dice
1 tbsp roughly chopped coriander
salt and freshly ground black pepper

Place the swordfish in a single layer in a shallow ceramic bowl. Mix together the lemon zest and juice, chilli flakes, mint and garlic. Spoon this over the fish and season well with sea salt. Cover and chill in the fridge for 20–30 minutes.

Preheat the oven to 200°C/Gas 6 and line a baking tray with non-stick baking parchment. Transfer the swordfish steaks to the baking tray, place in the oven and cook for 10–12 minutes or until the fish is just cooked through, taking care not to overcook it.

Mix all the salsa ingredients together in a bowl, season well with salt and freshly ground black pepper and divide between four plates. Top each serving with the baked swordfish and serve immediately.

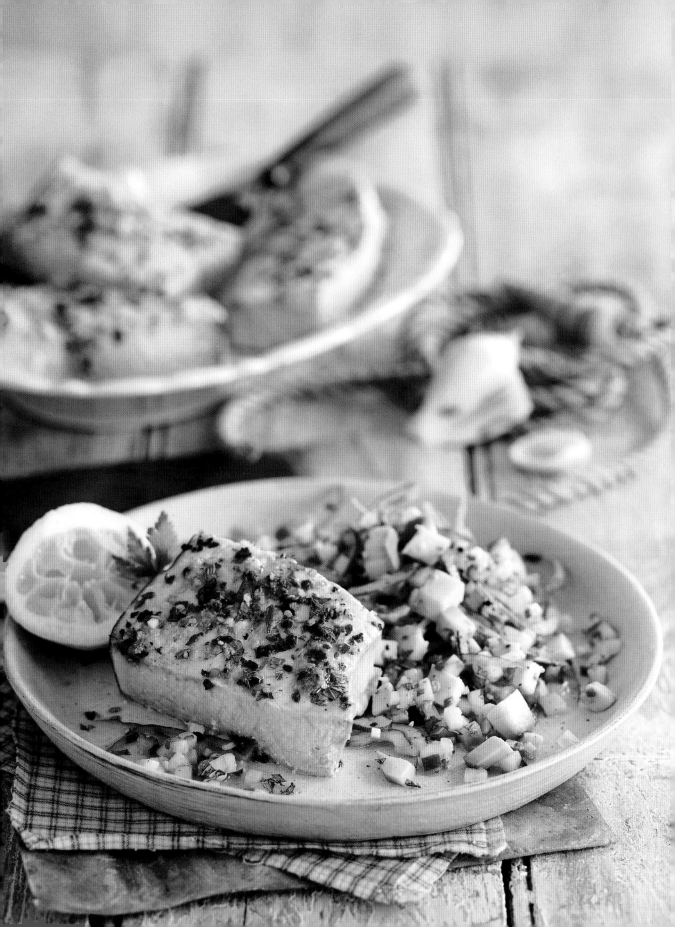

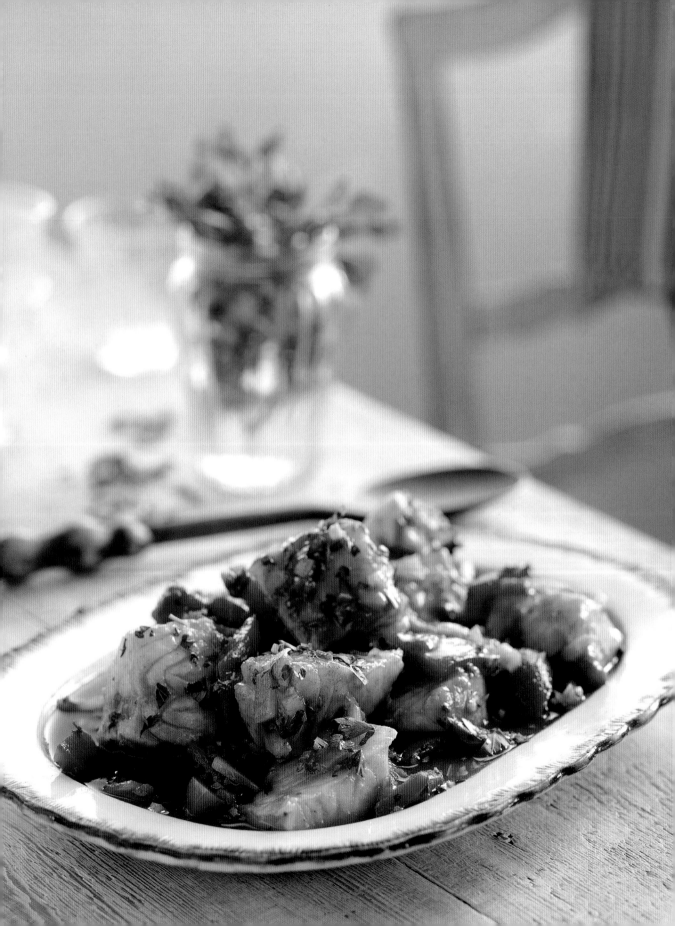

Ligurian fish stew

SERVES 4

EASY ✳

Syns per serving
Extra Easy: Free
Original: Free
Green: 5 Syns

Preparation time: 20 minutes
Cooking time: under 30 minutes

2 garlic cloves, peeled and crushed
1 small fennel bulb, trimmed and
finely chopped
1 tsp ground cumin
1 tsp paprika
1 tsp fennel seeds
a pinch of saffron threads
200ml/7fl oz fish stock
200g canned chopped tomatoes
1 red pepper, deseeded and
cut into 1cm/½in pieces
500g/1lb 2oz thick white fish fillets,
skinned and cut into large pieces
roughly chopped flat-leaf parsley,
to garnish

This fish stew is the perfect family feast. A well-flavoured base broth, including saffron and fennel seeds, is essential.

Put the garlic and fennel in a large saucepan and place over a low heat. Stir and cook gently for 4–5 minutes.

Add the cumin, paprika, fennel seeds and saffron threads and cook for 1 minute.

Add the stock and the tomatoes. Bring to the boil and then reduce the heat to medium. Add the red pepper and simmer for 8–10 minutes. Add the fish and simmer for 5 minutes.

Remove from the heat and ladle into soup bowls. Garnish with the parsley and serve immediately.

Tip For a luxurious version, add 100ml/3½fl oz white wine (add 1 Syn per serving) when you add the stock and tomatoes.

Roasted sea bass with basil and roasted vine tomatoes

SERVES 4

EASY

Syns per serving
Extra Easy: Free
Original: Free
Green: 25½ Syns

Preparation time: 15 minutes
Cooking time: about 30–35 minutes

1 whole sea bass (about 2kg/4lb 8oz),
gutted and scaled
salt and freshly ground black pepper
2 large lemons, thinly sliced
3 garlic cloves, peeled and crushed
a handful of basil, roughly chopped
400g/14oz vine tomatoes

Baking a whole fish is a good way of keeping it succulent, while imparting extra flavour at the same time. You can try other white fish like sea bream, hake or haddock for this recipe, if desired.

Preheat the oven to 220°C/Gas 7 and line a heavy baking sheet with non-stick baking parchment. Pat the sea bass dry, inside and out, with kitchen paper and season inside and out.

Lay three-quarters of the lemon slices on the baking sheet and place the fish on top. Carefully stuff the fish with the remaining lemon, the garlic and the basil.

Roast the fish in the oven for 15 minutes, then add the vine tomatoes around the fish and continue to roast for 15–20 minutes or until the fish is cooked through and the tomatoes are lightly roasted.

To serve, gently peel the fish skin back, then lift off a piece of the back fillet and a piece of the belly to make one serving: each side should yield two portions. Serve the sea bass immediately with the roast tomatoes.

Tuna al cartoccio

SERVES 4

EASY

Syns per serving
Extra Easy: ½ Syn
Original: ½ Syn
Green: 14 Syns

Preparation time: 15 minutes
Cooking time: under 15 minutes

4 x 200g/7oz tuna fillets
6 garlic cloves, peeled and roughly chopped
2 small dried red chillies, crumbled (or to taste)
a few rosemary sprigs
sea salt
2 tbsp dry white wine
4 tbsp chopped parsley, to serve
lemon wedges, to serve

Tuna has a wonderful, clean flavour and cooking it in baking parchment works brilliantly. The parchment lets the fish steam in its own juices while absorbing the aromas of the garlic, herbs and wine.

Preheat the oven to 220°C/Gas 7.

Place a large piece of aluminium foil, about 60cm/24in long, onto a work surface and cover with a layer of baking parchment almost the same size. Fold over the edges so that the foil and parchment are secured together at the edges.

Place the tuna fillets onto the parchment paper and scatter over the garlic, dried chillies and some rosemary leaves. Season with sea salt and pour over the wine.

Seal the parchment paper and foil around the fish fillets. Start at the ends, rolling the foil inwards to ensure the ends are properly sealed, then crimp the sides to create a pasty-shaped parcel. The parcel should be tightly sealed so the fish steams as it cooks without any steam escaping.

Place the fish in a roasting tray and put in the oven to roast for 10–12 minutes or until just cooked through.

When cooked, remove from the oven and place on a large serving plate. Carefully undo the foil and parchment, folding back the sides.

To serve, sprinkle with the chopped parsley and squeeze over fresh lemon juice.

Grilled mackerel with rosemary and garlic

SERVES 4

EASY

Syns per serving
Extra Easy: ½ Syn
Original: ½ Syn
Green: 22½ Syns

Preparation time: 15 minutes
Cooking time: 5–7 minutes

4 whole mackerel, heads removed,
gutted and cleaned
2 red chillies, deseeded and finely
chopped
2 garlic cloves, peeled and finely
chopped
salt and freshly ground black pepper
low calorie cooking spray
juice of 1 lemon
4 spring onions, trimmed and finely
sliced
4 tsp dried red chilli flakes
1 tbsp finely chopped rosemary
juice of 2 oranges
mixed salad leaves, to serve

Fish like mackerel are very popular throughout Italy. This isn't surprising, really, as mackerel are abundant along the extensive and beautiful Italian coastline.

Make four or five cuts on each side of each mackerel and sprinkle the red chillies and garlic into each cut.

Season with salt and pepper and spray each fish, on both sides, with low calorie cooking spray.

Preheat the grill or barbecue and, when hot, cook the fish for 5–7 minutes on each side or until the skin is crisp and lightly charred at the edges and the fish is just tender.

While the fish is under the grill, combine the lemon juice, spring onions, dried chilli flakes, rosemary and orange juice in a small bowl.

Drizzle the rosemary mixture over the mackerel and serve straight from the grill with a crisp mixed leaf salad.

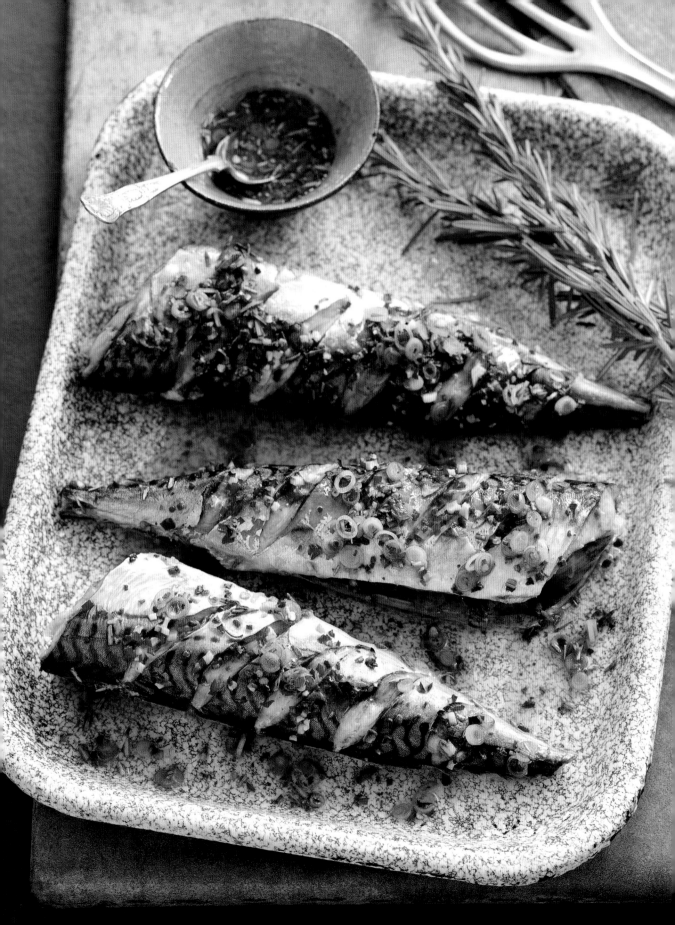

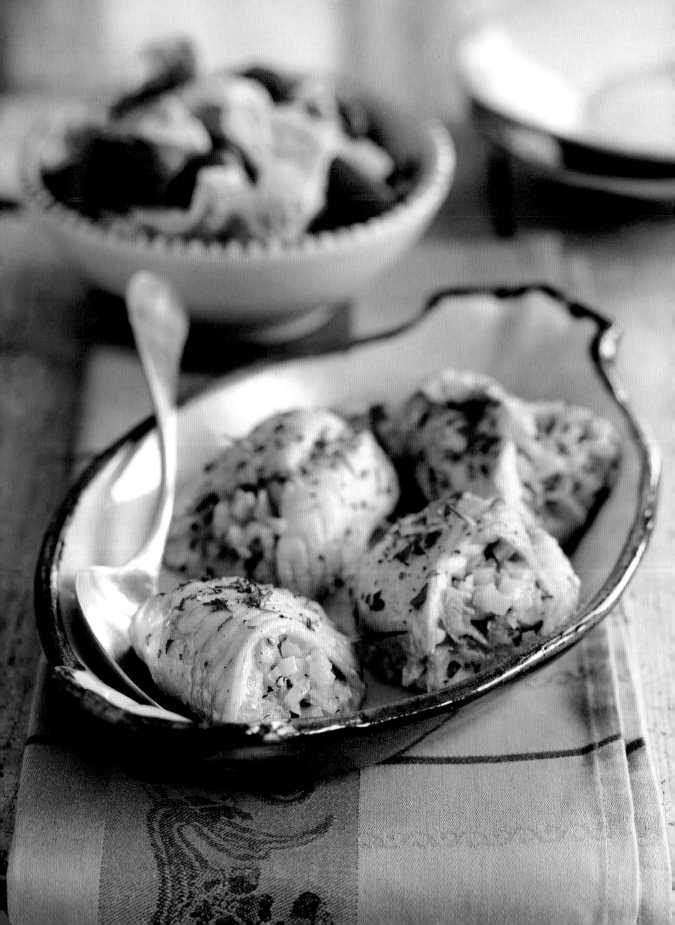

Stuffed salmon rolls with white wine and lemon

Stuffed with a fresh fennel, garlic and lemon filling, these tasty salmon rolls are surprisingly light. This recipe works equally well with any other firm-fleshed fish.

SERVES 4

WORTH THE EFFORT ❄ (if fish not previously frozen)

Syns per serving
Extra Easy: 1 Syn
Original: 1 Syn
Green: 14 Syns

Preparation time: 25 minutes
Cooking time: under 30 minutes

4 x 150g/5oz salmon fillets, skinned
salt and freshly ground black pepper
125ml/4½fl oz dry white wine
2 tbsp finely chopped flat-leaf parsley
crisp salad leaves, to serve
tomato wedges, to serve

FOR THE STUFFING
60ml/2fl oz fish stock
1 small fennel bulb, trimmed and finely chopped
1 garlic clove, peeled and crushed
finely grated zest of 1 lemon

Make the stuffing by placing the fish stock, fennel and garlic into a saucepan and bringing it to the boil. Reduce the heat to low, cover and simmer gently for 10 minutes, stirring often. Remove from the heat and stir in the lemon zest.

Meanwhile, lay the salmon fillets in a single layer on a work surface and cover with cling film. Lightly beat with a wooden mallet or rolling pin until they are as thin as possible without breaking them. Remove the cling film and season well.

Preheat the oven to 190°C/Gas 5.

Divide the stuffing mixture between the flattened fillets. Roll up the fish and secure with cocktail sticks. Place the stuffed fish in a single layer in a shallow ovenproof dish and pour over the wine. Scatter over the parsley and bake in the oven for 12–15 minutes or until the fish is cooked through.

Remove from the oven and serve immediately with the salad leaves and tomatoes.

Italian bacon-wrapped monkfish

SERVES 4

EASY ✱ (if fish not previously frozen)

Syns per serving
Extra Easy: Free
Original: Free
Green: 12½ Syns

Preparation time: 10 minutes
Cooking time: about 10 minutes

finely grated zest and juice of 1 lemon
8 tbsp finely chopped flat-leaf parsley
4 garlic cloves, peeled and
finely chopped
1 tbsp quark
salt and freshly ground black pepper
4 x 200g/7oz monkfish tail fillets
12 rashers of lean bacon, all visible fat
removed and stretched with the back
of a knife

The bacon flavours the delicate flesh of the monkfish in this recipe while protecting it from the heat of the pan so that it remains moist and tender. You can also cook the fish over a barbecue or under the grill if you prefer.

Place the lemon zest and juice, parsley, garlic and quark in a bowl and stir until well mixed. Season well with salt and pepper.

Place the monkfish on a work surface and, using a sharp knife, make a deep incision about 6cm/2½in long in the side of each fillet.

Stuff each fillet with the lemon mixture and then carefully wrap 3 bacon rashers around each one to enclose completely. Secure with a cocktail stick.

Heat a large non-stick frying pan over a high heat and when hot add the fish and cook for 4–5 minutes on each side or until just cooked through and the bacon is crispy.

Remove from the heat and allow to rest for 1–2 minutes before serving. The wrapped monkfish is delicious served with spinach and Rosemary Roasties (see page 120).

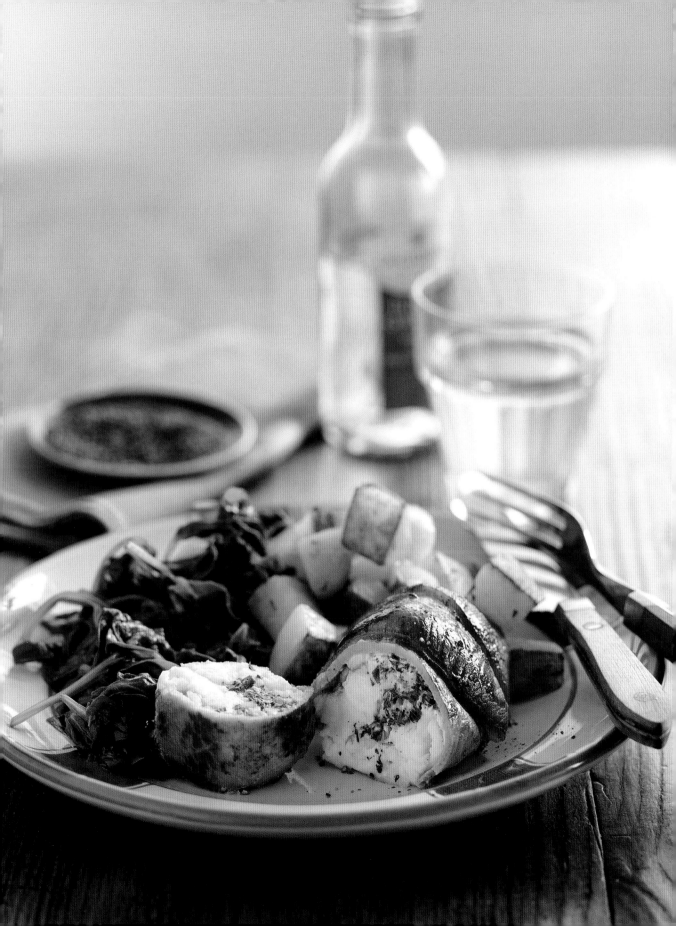

Red mullet with thyme in vine leaves

SERVES 4

EASY ✻ (if fish not previously frozen)

Syns per serving
Extra Easy: Free
Original: Free
Green: 19½ Syns

Preparation time: 20 minutes
Cooking time: about 10 minutes

4 x 350g/12oz red mullet, cleaned,
gutted and scaled
salt and freshly ground black pepper
4 tbsp roughly chopped thyme
2 tbsp finely grated lemon zest
1 tbsp peeled and finely chopped garlic
2 tsp finely chopped red chilli
4 large vine leaves in brine, rinsed and
patted dry
lemon wedges, to serve

Vine leaves, preserved in brine, are available in packets or jars – make sure you rinse them thoroughly in cold water before use. Wrapping the fish in vine leaves protects the delicate flesh and keeps it moist, sealing in all the lovely flavours.

Place the mullet on a work surface and season well with salt and pepper.

Mix together the thyme, lemon zest, garlic and red chilli in a bowl and use this mixture to stuff the fish.

Preheat the grill to medium-hot or a barbecue to medium. Wrap each fish tightly in a vine leaf, leaving the head and tails exposed, and place on a grill rack. Cook under the grill or over the barbecue for 3–4 minutes on each side or until cooked through.

Remove from the grill rack and place on a serving plate. Remove and discard the vine leaves and serve with wedges of lemon to squeeze over.

Prawns in tomato, courgette and basil sauce

SERVES 4

EASY

Syns per serving
Extra Easy: Free
Original: Free
Green: 7½ Syns

Preparation time: 10 minutes
Cooking time: 30–35 minutes

800g/1lb 12oz raw, peeled tiger prawns
salt and freshly ground black pepper
low calorie cooking spray
1 onion, peeled and finely chopped
2 garlic cloves, peeled and crushed
1 tsp dried red chilli flakes
5 tbsp roughly chopped basil
2 x 400g cans chopped tomatoes
1 courgette, cut into 1cm/½in dice

If you want to wow your guests, serve this dish at a summer dinner party – it's bursting with the flavours of the sea and sun.

Place the prawns in a ceramic bowl and season well with salt and pepper.

Spray a wide saucepan with low calorie cooking spray, place over a low heat and cook the onion and garlic for 4–5 minutes or until softened.

Add the chilli flakes, basil, tomatoes and courgette and cook over a medium-low heat for 20 minutes or until you have a thick sauce. Season well.

Increase the heat to high and bring the mixture to the boil. Stir in the prawns and cook for 6–8 minutes or until the prawns turn pink and are cooked through.

Remove from the heat and serve immediately.

Gamberini al cartoccio

SERVES 4

EASY ✱ (if prawns not previously
frozen)

Syns per serving
Extra Easy: Free
Original: Free
Green: 10 Syns

Preparation time: 25 minutes
Cooking time: about 20 minutes

6 spring onions, trimmed and
roughly chopped
1 fennel bulb, trimmed and finely sliced
200g/7oz green beans, trimmed and
cut into 3cm/1¼in lengths
6 midi plum tomatoes, quartered
4 tbsp lemon juice
1 tsp crushed dried red chilli flakes
2 tsp dried oregano
4 garlic cloves, peeled and sliced
1kg/2lb 4oz raw king or
tiger prawns, peeled
salt and freshly ground black pepper
chopped dill or fennel fronds,
to garnish

Baking prawns in sealed paper parcels is an excellent way of retaining their delicate flavour and enticing aroma as they cook.

Preheat the oven to 240°C/Gas 9 and cut out four 50cm/20in squares of foil or baking parchment.

In a large bowl, mix the spring onions and fennel with the green beans, tomatoes, lemon juice, chilli flakes, oregano and garlic.

Place a quarter of the vegetable mixture onto the centre of each piece of foil or parchment.

Divide the prawns between the pieces of foil or parchment and season well.

Bring the edges of the foil or parchment together to form a loose parcel around the prawns. Seal the edges by folding tightly and place the parcels on two large baking trays.

Bake in the oven for 15–20 minutes. Transfer the parcels to serving plates and leave to stand for 5 minutes. Split the parcels open, garnish with the dill or fennel fronds and serve immediately.

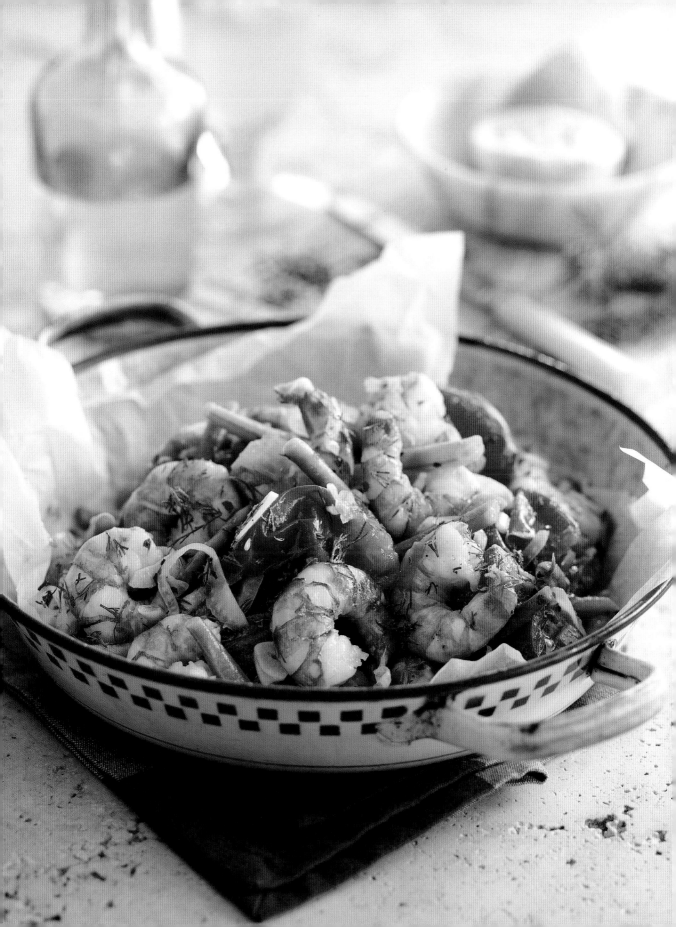

Italian-style mixed seafood grill

Syns per serving
Extra Easy: Free
Original: Free
Green: 13½ Syns

Preparation time: 10 minutes
Cooking time: under 20 minutes

1kg/2lb 4oz mixed fish fillets (brill, coley, cod, red mullet, sea bream), cut into large pieces
sea salt and freshly ground black pepper
12 mussels, cleaned
12 clams, cleaned
12 large raw prawns, in their shell

FOR THE DRESSING
finely grated zest and juice of 1 lemon
1 tbsp capers, rinsed
1 shallot, peeled and finely chopped
4 tbsp finely chopped flat-leaf parsley
2 garlic cloves, peeled and crushed
a pinch of dried chilli flakes
200ml/7fl oz fat free vinaigrette

This vibrant seafood meal depends on the freshest fish for its success. You can use any seasonal fish you can find.

Preheat the oven to 190°C/Gas 5, or preheat the grill until hot.

Season the fish fillets well and place on a baking tray in the oven or under the grill and cook for 6–8 minutes or until cooked through. Remove from the heat, cover and set aside.

Place the shellfish on a baking tray in a single layer and cook for 6–8 minutes or until the clams and mussels have opened, discarding any that remain closed, and the prawns have turned pink and are cooked through. Remove from the heat, cover and keep warm.

Make the dressing by mixing all the ingredients together in a bowl. Season well.

To serve, place all the seafood on a large platter and drizzle over the dressing. Have finger bowls of warm water alongside to clean your hands as you eat.

Griddled squid salad with mint and coriander

Fresh squid is available from all good fishmongers and the fish counters in most supermarkets. Here it makes a delectable main when combined with the Italian fresh herb sauce salsa verde.

SERVES 4

EASY

Syns per serving
Extra Easy: Free
Original: Free
Green: 8 Syns

Preparation time: 20 minutes plus marinating
Cooking time: 10–12 minutes

800g/1lb 12oz squid, cleaned
finely grated zest and juice of 2 limes
1 red chilli, deseeded and finely diced
1 tsp sea salt
1 garlic clove, peeled and crushed

FOR THE SALSA VERDE
4 spring onions, trimmed and very finely chopped
4 tbsp finely chopped flat-leaf parsley
4 tbsp finely chopped mint
2 garlic cloves, peeled and crushed
2 tbsp capers, rinsed
100ml/3½fl oz fat free vinaigrette

Place the squid on a clean work surface and make a cut down one side of the body tube and open it. Using a sharp knife, lightly score the inside of the flesh in a criss-cross pattern, which will help tenderise it, then cut the squid into bite-sized pieces.

Mix the lime zest, red chilli, sea salt and garlic together in a small bowl and rub into the squid and leave to marinate for 2–3 hours in the fridge.

Meanwhile, make the salsa verde by mixing all the ingredients together in a bowl along with the lime juice. Set aside.

Heat a non-stick ridged griddle until smoking hot. Remove the squid from the marinade with a slotted spoon and cook on each side for no more than 2 minutes or it will become tough, pushing the squid down onto the griddle with the back of a fish slice.

Remove the squid from the heat and serve with the salsa verde spooned over.

Mussels in herb and tomato sauce

SERVES 4

EASY

Syns per serving
Extra Easy: 4 Syns
Green: 7½ Syns
Original: 18½ Syns

Preparation time: 10 minutes
Cooking time: about 20 minutes

low calorie cooking spray
4 shallots, peeled and finely chopped
3 garlic cloves, peeled and crushed
2 tsp dried oregano
6 tbsp roughly chopped
flat-leaf parsley
400g can chopped cherry tomatoes
2 level tbsp sun-dried tomato purée
salt and freshly ground black pepper
1kg/2lb 4oz fresh mussels
350g/12oz dried tagliatelle
50g/2oz Parmesan cheese, grated
basil leaves, to garnish

Mussels cooked in a herby tomato sauce are a marriage made in heaven. Be sure to have finger bowls of warm water with lemon on the table so that you can clean your hands while you eat.

Spray a wide saucepan with low calorie cooking spray, place over a low heat and cook the shallots and garlic for 4–5 minutes or until they have softened.

Add the oregano, parsley, tomatoes and tomato purée and cook over a medium-low heat for 12–15 minutes or until you have a thick sauce. Season well.

While the sauce is cooking, place the mussels in a bowl of cold water, discarding any that are open or broken. Scrub them with a brush and remove any 'beards'.

Increase the heat under the saucepan to high and bring the mixture to the boil. Add the mussels, cover and cook for 5–6 minutes, shaking the pan from time to time, until all the mussels have opened and are cooked through (discard any mussels that remain closed).

Meanwhile, cook the pasta according to the packet instructions and drain well. Transfer to a serving bowl and ladle over the mussel mixture.

Sprinkle over the Parmesan cheese and basil leaves before serving.

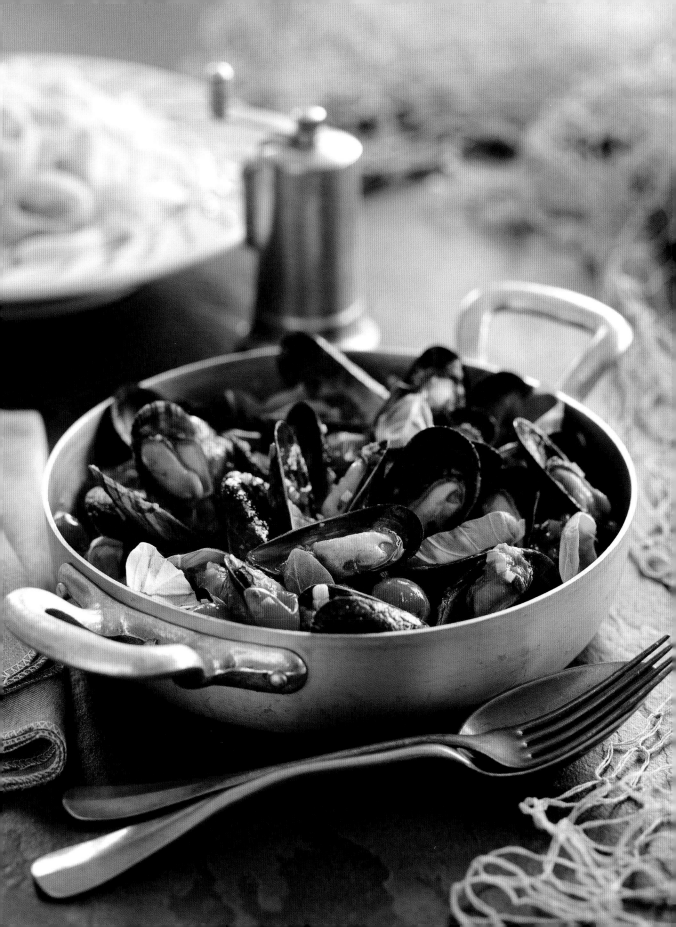

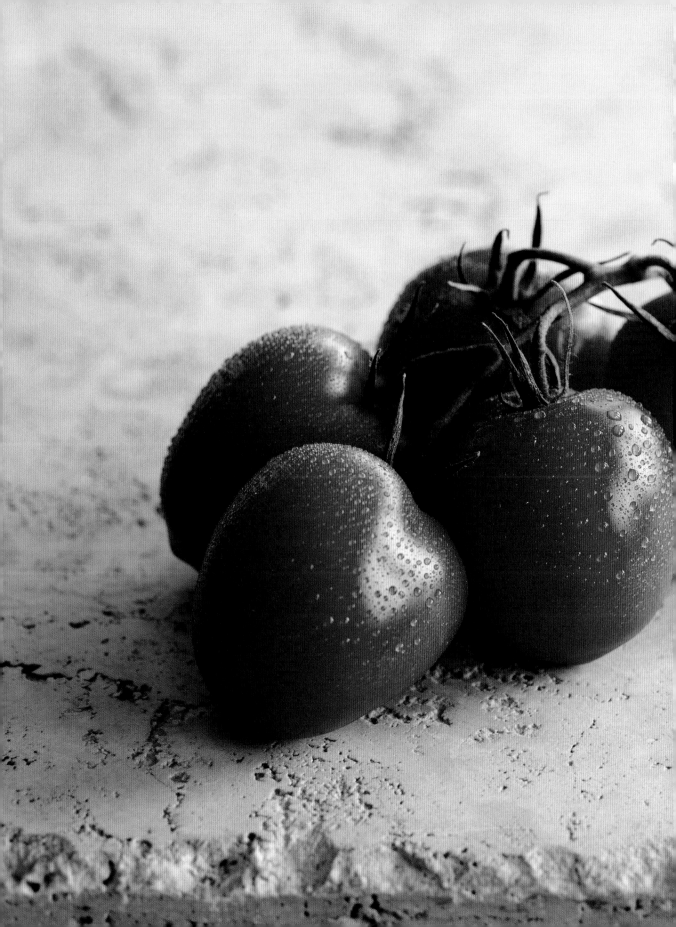

Chapter 5

Meat and poultry

Our selection of meat and poultry dishes includes restaurant classics like Osso Bucco, a melt-in-the-mouth slow-cooked veal stew (see page 150), and Bistecca alla Pizzaiola – a juicy steak topped with a lively sauce of tomatoes and garlic (see page 151). As well as hearty, savoury casseroles, Italian main courses often feature meat grilled simply, such as lamb cutlets spiked with rosemary and lemon, or pork chops topped with red pesto. From quick family suppers to special-occasion dinners, eating Italian-style always has plenty of delicious choices to offer.

Pollo alla diavola

SERVES 4

EASY ⊛

Syns per serving
Extra Easy: Free
Original: Free
Green: 15 Syns

Preparation time: 20 minutes
Cooking time: under 20 minutes

8 skinless chicken breast fillets
finely grated zest and juice of 4 lemons
2 red chillies, deseeded and very finely chopped
4 garlic cloves, peeled and crushed
2–3 tsp crushed dried red chilli flakes
salt
low calorie cooking spray
chopped flat-leaf parsley, to garnish
lemon wedges, to garnish

Pollo alla diavola or 'devil's-style chicken' is an intensely flavoured dish. Just reduce the quantity of chilli if you prefer something milder.

Lay the chicken fillets on a clean work surface between two sheets of cling film. Then flatten the fillets with a meat mallet or rolling pin until they are about 1cm/½in thick. Remove the cling film and place the chicken in a single layer in a wide, shallow ceramic dish.

Mix together the lemon zest and juice, red chillies, garlic and dried chilli flakes and season well with salt. Pour this mixture over the chicken, cover and leave to marinate for at least 2–4 hours (or overnight if time permits).

When ready to cook, preheat the grill to medium-hot. Remove the chicken from the marinade and place on a rack over a baking sheet, spray with low calorie cooking spray and cook the chicken under the grill for 6–8 minutes on each side or until cooked through.

Remove from the grill and serve garnished with the chopped parsley and the lemon wedges to squeeze over.

Chicken, sage and pancetta skewers

SERVES 4

EASY ✳

Syns per serving
Extra Easy: 3 Syns
Original: 3 Syns
Green: 11½ Syns

Preparation time: 20 minutes
Cooking time: 12–15 minutes

12 slices pancetta, cut into
bite-sized pieces
3 skinless chicken breast fillets,
cut into bite-sized pieces
8 large mushrooms, quartered
1 large red onion, peeled and
cut into wedges
1 courgette, cut into chunky rounds
4 sage leaves
low calorie cooking spray
salt and freshly ground black pepper
a crisp green salad, to serve

You can use turkey breast instead of chicken in this recipe if you'd like a change.

Preheat the grill to medium-high.

Thread the pancetta, chicken and vegetables onto four long metal skewers, adding a sage leaf to each one.

Spray with low calorie cooking spray and cook under the grill for 12–15 minutes, turning occasionally or until the chicken and vegetables are cooked and the pancetta is crisp.

Season well and serve with the green salad.

Chicken involtini

SERVES 4

WORTH THE EFFORT ❄

Syns per serving
Extra Easy: 1½ Syns
Original: 1½ Syns
Green: 10½ Syns

Preparation time: 25 minutes
Cooking time: 20–25 minutes

1 small carrot, peeled and cut into
finger-length thin strips
50g/2oz green beans, trimmed
4 skinless chicken breast fillets
salt and freshly ground black pepper
4 tbsp fat free onion and chive
cottage cheese
2 garlic cloves, peeled and crushed
2 tsp dried basil
2 tsp finely grated lemon zest
4 slices of Parma ham
low calorie cooking spray
3 tbsp dry Marsala wine

Parma ham, one of many Italian cured meats, is used in this rolled, stuffed chicken dish. It enriches, moisturises and imparts a wonderful flavour to the chicken.

Preheat the oven to 190°C/Gas 5.

Blanch the carrot and green beans in a pan of lightly salted boiling water for 1–2 minutes. Drain and set aside.

Place each chicken breast between two pieces of cling film and pound with a meat mallet or rolling pin to roughly make a 10 x 16cm/4 x 6½in thin piece. Season lightly.

Mix together the cottage cheese with the garlic, basil and lemon zest in a bowl.

Cover each chicken breast with a slice of Parma ham and then spread each with the cottage cheese mixture. Mix together the carrot and green beans and divide between the flattened breasts.

Roll up each chicken breast tightly and tie at each end with kitchen string or secure with a couple of cocktail sticks.

Place in an ovenproof frying pan and spray lightly with low calorie cooking spray. Drizzle over the Marsala wine and cook for 20–25 minutes or until the chicken is cooked through and the vegetables are tender. Serve immediately.

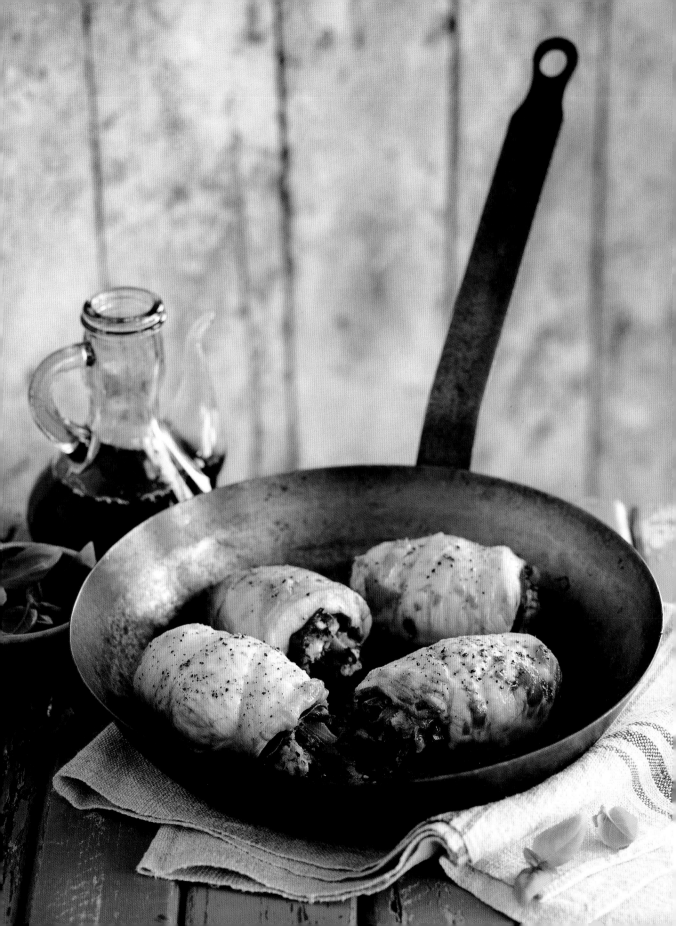

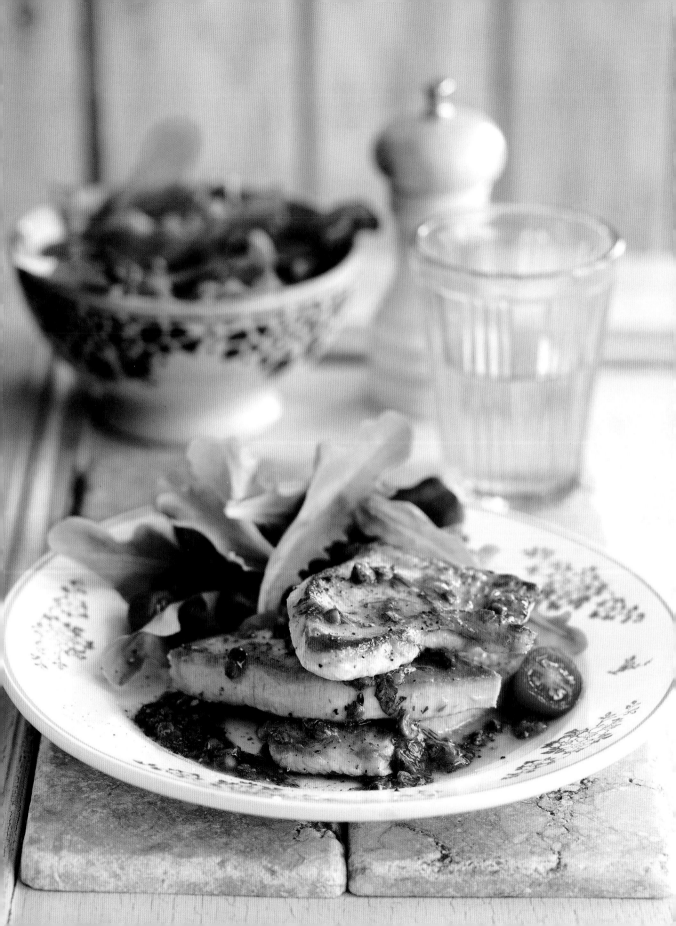

Piccata al limone

SERVES 4

EASY ❄

Syns per serving
Extra Easy: Free
Original: Free
Green: 5½ Syns

Preparation time: 15 minutes
Cooking time: under 20 minutes

4 skinless and boneless
turkey breast steaks
salt and freshly ground black pepper
low calorie cooking spray
250ml/9fl oz chicken stock
2 tbsp rinsed and chopped capers
1 tbsp fresh lemon juice
4 tbsp chopped Italian or
flat-leaf parsley
mixed salad leaves, to serve
halved cherry tomatoes, to serve

Traditionally made with veal escalopes, here we use thin turkey breast steaks for this delicious yet simple Italian recipe.

Place the turkey steaks between two sheets of cling film. Then use a meat mallet or rolling pin to pound them to a 5mm/¼in thickness. Season well.

Spray the turkey steaks with low calorie cooking spray. Heat a large non-stick frying pan sprayed with low calorie cooking spray and place over a high heat. Add the steaks to the pan and cook for 5–6 minutes on each side or until nicely browned.

Pour the chicken stock into the pan and allow to boil for 5–6 minutes over a high heat. Stir in the capers, lemon juice and parsley.

Remove from the heat and serve immediately with the salad leaves and tomatoes.

Roasted duck breasts with Parma ham

SERVES 4

EASY

Syns per serving
Extra Easy: 1 Syn
Original: 1 Syn
Green: 17½ Syns

Preparation time: 15–20 minutes
Cooking time: 20–25 minutes

4 skinless duck breast fillets
2 garlic cloves, peeled and crushed
3 tbsp finely chopped tarragon
or parsley
2 tbsp fat free natural cottage cheese
4 tsp finely grated lemon zest,
plus extra to garnish
1 tsp dried chilli flakes (optional)
salt and freshly ground black pepper
8 thin slices of Parma ham
griddled courgettes and aubergines,
to serve
lemon wedges, to garnish

Duck breasts are stuffed with a herb and lemon mixture and then wrapped in slices of Parma ham to impart flavour and keep them moist while cooking.

Preheat the oven to 220°C/Gas 7. Using a small sharp knife, make a cut down each duck breast to make a 'pocket'.

Mix the garlic, tarragon or parsley, cottage cheese, lemon zest and dried chilli flakes, if using, in a small bowl until well combined. Season well.

Stuff the duck breasts with this mixture, carefully wrap each breast with 2 slices of the ham and secure with a cocktail stick.

Place on a baking tray and cook in the oven for 20–25 minutes or until the Parma ham is lightly browned and the duck is cooked through.

Remove from the oven and serve immediately with griddled courgettes and aubergines and garnished with lemon wedges.

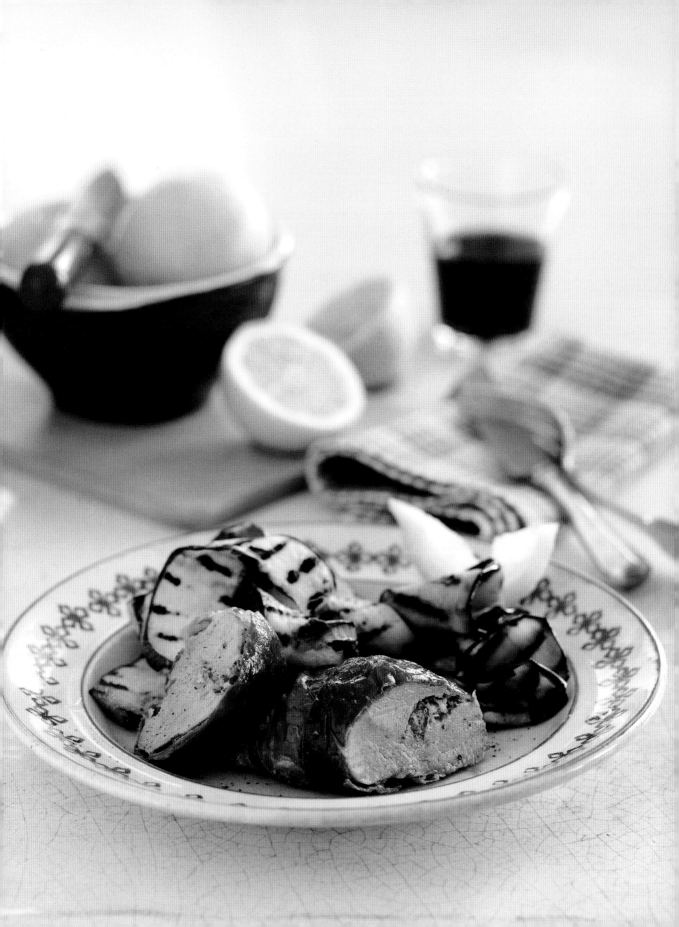

Balsamic vinegar poached poussins

SERVES 4

EASY ❄

Syns per serving
Extra Easy: ½ Syn
Original: ½ Syn
Green: 11½ Syns

Preparation time: 15 minutes
plus marinating
Cooking time: about 1½ hours

4 x 300g poussins
finely grated zest and juice
of 2 oranges
4 garlic cloves, peeled and crushed
6 tbsp balsamic vinegar
800ml/28fl oz chicken stock
2 carrots, peeled and roughly chopped
2 celery sticks, roughly chopped
3 small onions, peeled and halved

Balsamic vinegar adds a wonderful flavour to the poussins in this simple rustic dish from Italy.

Place the poussins in a single layer in a deep, ceramic dish.

Mix the orange zest and juice, garlic and balsamic vinegar in a small bowl. Pour over the poussins and turn to coat evenly. Cover and marinate them in the fridge for 6–8 hours (or overnight if time permits).

Preheat the oven to 160°C/Gas 3.

Place the poussins in a large heavy-based casserole dish and pour over the stock. Add the carrots, celery and onion, bring to the boil and cover with a lid. Then put in the oven and cook for 1½ hours or until the poussins are meltingly tender.

Remove the skin from the poussins and place them in wide shallow bowls. Spoon over the vegetables and stock and serve immediately.

Stuffed grilled lamb cutlets

SERVES 4

WORTH THE EFFORT ❄

Syns per serving
Extra Easy: Free
Original: Free
Green: 11½ Syns

Preparation time: 25 minutes
Cooking time: under 12–16 minutes

12 lean lamb cutlets
steamed vegetables or a mixed salad,
to serve

FOR THE FILLING
10 fresh sage leaves
2 tbsp finely chopped rosemary
4 tbsp finely chopped parsley
5 tbsp finely chopped basil
2 garlic cloves, peeled and
finely chopped
juice of 1 lemon
salt and freshly ground black pepper

Mixed herbs, garlic and lemon flavour these delicious cutlets and turn them into a special treat.

For the filling, place all the chopped herbs in a bowl with the garlic and lemon juice, season and mix well until you have a fairly smooth mixture.

Slice each lamb cutlet horizontally through the centre, leaving it joined at one end, and open it up like a butterfly. Lay the cutlets in a single layer on a work surface and cover with cling film. Lightly beat with a meat mallet or rolling pin to flatten the cutlets.

Spread the herb mixture on one side of each cutlet and fold the other side over the top to make a herby sandwich. Press together, making sure that none of the filling escapes.

Preheat the grill to hot and line a baking tray with foil. Transfer the cutlets to the baking tray and season to taste.

Place under the grill and cook for about 3–4 minutes on each side for rare, 4–5 minutes for medium or 6–8 minutes for well-done.

Serve immediately with the steamed vegetables or mixed salad.

Florentine lamb and vegetable stew

SERVES 4

EASY ✻

Syns per serving
Extra Easy: Free
Original: Free
Green: 19½ Syns

Preparation time: 20 minutes
Cooking time: about 1½ hours

1kg/2lb 4oz lean lamb steaks,
cut into bite-sized pieces
4 celery sticks, roughly chopped
3 carrots, peeled and
cut into large pieces
1 bay leaf
1 tsp Italian herb seasoning
20 baby onions, peeled but left whole
1.25 litres/2 pints lamb stock
salt and freshly ground black pepper
chopped flat-leaf parsley, to garnish

This is a fine, robust dish that will almost cook itself and is a great dish for hassle-free entertaining.

Place the lamb in a heavy-based casserole dish. Add the celery, carrots, bay leaf, Italian seasoning, baby onions and lamb stock. Season well and bring the mixture to the boil.

Cover tightly, reduce the heat to low and cook over a low heat for 1½ hours or until the lamb is meltingly tender.

Remove from the heat and garnish with chopped parsley before serving.

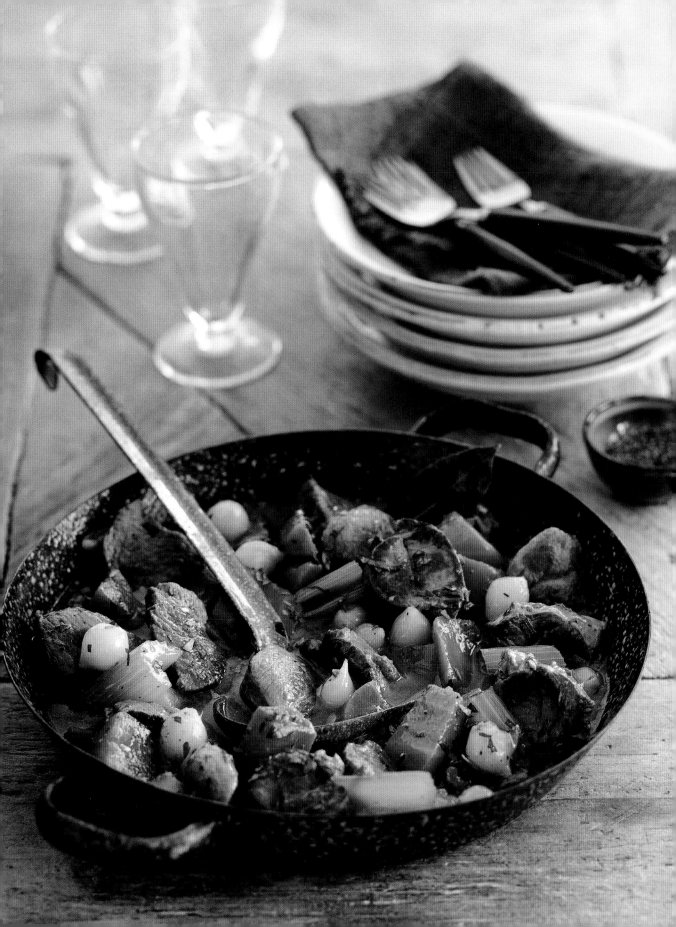

Sardinian lamb and fennel casserole

SERVES 4

EASY ✳

Syns per serving
Extra Easy: Free
Original: Free
Green: 19½ Syns

Preparation time: 15 minutes
Cooking time: about 1½ hours

1kg/2lb 4oz lean lamb steaks,
cut into bite-sized pieces
2 onions, peeled and thinly sliced
2 garlic cloves, peeled and chopped
2 x 400g cans chopped tomatoes
2 tsp dried oregano
2 fennel bulbs, trimmed and cut into
slices, reserving the fronds
salt and freshly ground black pepper

Wild fennel grows prolifically in Sardinia and the rugged countryside is sheep country, so the wonderful combination of ingredients in this delicious stew is a match made in heaven!

Place the lamb in a heavy-based casserole dish. Add the onions, garlic and tomatoes to the dish and sprinkle over the oregano.

Add the fennel to the lamb mixture, season well and bring the mixture to the boil.

Cover tightly, reduce the heat to low and cook over a low heat for 1½ hours or until the lamb is meltingly tender.

Just before serving, finely chop the fennel fronds and scatter over.

Sicilian-style meatballs in tomato sauce

SERVES 4

WORTH THE EFFORT ✳

Syns per serving
Extra Easy: Free
Original: Free
Green: 9½ Syns

Preparation time: 25 minutes
Cooking time: under 45 minutes

FOR THE SAUCE
1 onion, peeled and finely chopped
2 garlic cloves, peeled and
finely chopped
2 x 400g cans chopped tomatoes
4 tbsp finely chopped basil

FOR THE MEATBALLS
600g/1lb 5oz extra lean minced beef
1 small onion, peeled and
finely chopped
2 garlic cloves, peeled and
grated or crushed
2 tsp dried oregano
1 tbsp fennel seeds
4 tbsp finely chopped basil
salt and freshly ground black pepper
1 small egg, lightly beaten
chopped parsley, to garnish

This hearty recipe makes for a great family meal and can be served with rice, pasta or potatoes, if desired.

First make the tomato sauce. Put all the sauce ingredients into a frying pan or saucepan and bring to the boil. Reduce the heat and simmer gently for 15–20 minutes, stirring often.

To make the meatballs, put the minced beef, onion, garlic, oregano, fennel seeds, basil and seasoning in a large bowl and mix well together. Bind with the beaten egg, and then divide into about 20 portions. Roll each one into a ball, using your hands.

Place a non-stick frying pan over a medium high heat. Brown the meatballs for 5–6 minutes and then remove with a slotted spoon.

Add the meatballs to the tomato sauce, cover and cook gently over a low heat for about 15 minutes, until the meat is thoroughly cooked.

Serve sprinkled with chopped parsley.

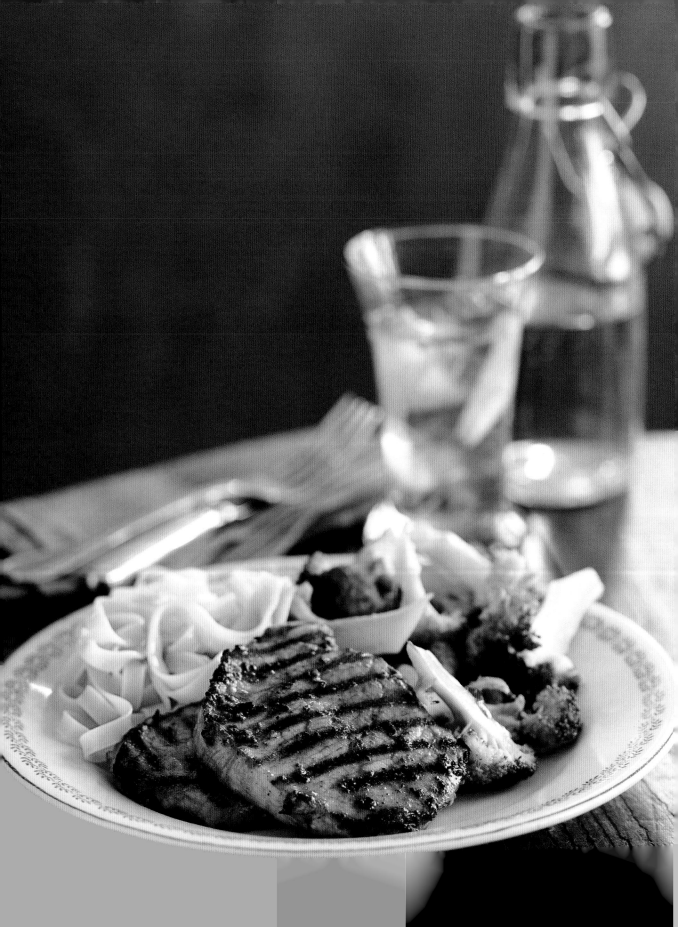

Grilled pork with red pesto

SERVES 4

WORTH THE EFFORT ✻

Syns per serving
Extra Easy: 1½ Syns
Original: 16 Syns
Green: 25½ Syns

Preparation time: 20 minutes plus
marinating
Cooking time: 10–12 minutes

8 lean pork loin steaks
2 garlic cloves, peeled and
very finely chopped
1 tbsp finely chopped sage
2 level tbsp red pesto
350g/12oz dried tagliatelle
salt and freshly ground black pepper

In this delicious recipe, beautifully lean pork steaks are marinated with a red pesto mixture to guarantee the chops are flavoursome all the way through.

Cut a horizontal pocket through the centre of each pork steak.

Mix together the garlic, sage and pesto in a small bowl and rub this mixture all over the outside and inside of the steaks. Place in a dish, cover and leave to marinate in the fridge for 4–6 hours (or overnight if time permits).

Cook the pasta according to the packet instructions. Drain well.

Meanwhile, preheat the grill to hot and line a baking sheet with foil. Season the outside and inside of the steaks, place them on the baking sheet lined with foil and cook under the grill, about 10cm/4in from the heat source, for 5–6 minutes on each side or until cooked through.

Remove from the grill and serve immediately with the tagliatelle and Broccoli with Chilli and Garlic (see page 185).

Northern Italian pot-roasted pork loin

SERVES 4–6

EASY ✳

Syns per serving (serves 4)
Extra Easy: 1 Syn
Original: 6½ Syns
Green: 24½ Syns

Syns per serving (serves 6)
Extra Easy: ½ Syn
Original: 4½ Syns
Green: 16½ Syns

Preparation time: 20 minutes
Cooking time: about 1½ hours

1 boned and rolled lean loin of pork
salt and freshly ground black pepper
2 celery sticks, finely chopped
1 onion, peeled and finely chopped
1 carrot, peeled and finely chopped
2 garlic cloves,
peeled and finely chopped
6 sage leaves
3 rosemary sprigs
100ml/3½fl oz dry white wine
2 tbsp juniper berries
400ml/14fl oz chicken or
vegetable stock
600g/1lb 5oz potatoes,
peeled and thickly sliced
low calorie cooking spray
300g/11oz green beans, halved

This rather grand dish from Northern Italy is perfect for lavish entertaining. The pork loin is roasted in a sauce flavoured with wine, juniper berries, rosemary and sage until it's meltingly tender.

Preheat the oven to 180°C/Gas 4. Season the pork loin well with salt and pepper and place in a heavy-based casserole dish.

Add the chopped vegetables, garlic, herbs, wine, juniper berries and stock. Bring the mixture to the boil, cover tightly, place in the oven and cook for 1½ hours or until the pork is meltingly tender.

Meanwhile, cook the potatoes in a saucepan of lightly salted boiling water for 7–8 minutes. Drain well. Spray a large non-stick frying pan with low calorie cooking spray, add the potatoes and stir-fry for 5–6 minutes until golden.

Blanch the green beans in a saucepan of lightly salted boiling water for 3–4 minutes. Drain well.

Remove the rind from the pork and carve into slices. Strain the cooking juices from the casserole. Serve the pork with the sautéed potatoes and green beans and the strained vegetables poured over.

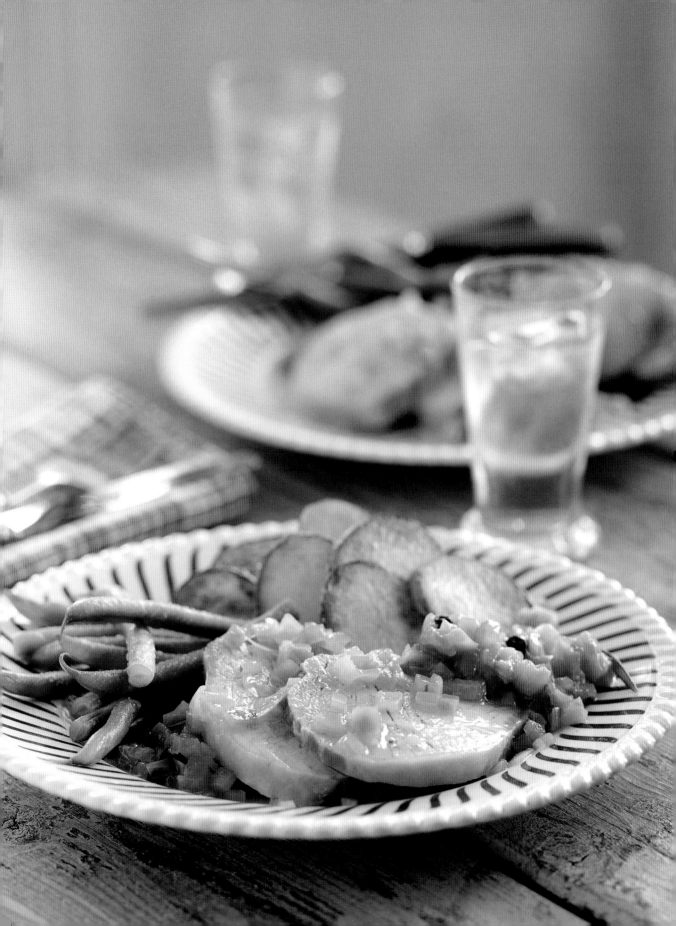

Osso bucco

SERVES 4

EASY ❋

Syns per serving
Extra Easy: Free
Original: Free
Green: 15 Syns

Preparation time: 10 minutes
Cooking time: about 2 hours

4 thickly sliced veal shanks with the
bone marrow and all visible
fat removed
3 garlic cloves, peeled and sliced
1 onion, peeled and finely chopped
2 carrots, peeled and finely chopped
4 celery sticks, finely chopped
1 bay leaf
400g can chopped tomatoes
600ml/21fl oz chicken stock
salt and freshly ground black pepper
chopped flat-leaf parsley, to garnish

This terrific dish of succulent veal cooked slowly is perfect for lazy entertaining as it's hassle free to make and, even better, almost cooks itself.

Preheat the oven to 160°C/Gas 3.

Place the meat in a large heavy-based casserole dish in a single layer.

Add the garlic, onion, carrots, celery, bay leaf and tomatoes and stock. Season well, bring to the boil, cover tightly and place in the oven for 2 hours or until the meat is meltingly tender.

Serve the veal topped with the vegetable sauce mixture and garnished with chopped parsley.

Bistecca alla pizzaiola

SERVES 4

EASY ✳

These delicious Italian-style beef steaks with tomato, garlic and herbs are sure to become a family favourite.

Syns per serving
Extra Easy: Free
Original: Free
Green: 14½ Syns

Preparation time: 10 minutes
Cooking time: 30–35 minutes

4 lean fillet steaks, all visible fat removed
salt and freshly ground black pepper
low calorie cooking spray
1 onion, peeled and finely chopped
2 garlic cloves, peeled and crushed
400g can chopped cherry tomatoes
1 tbsp dried oregano
4 tbsp roughly chopped basil
a wild rocket leaf salad, to serve

Season the steaks and place in a hot non-stick ridged griddle. Cook for 3–4 minutes on each side or until cooked to your liking, remove and keep warm.

Spray a large frying pan with low calorie cooking spray and place over a medium heat. Add the onion, garlic, tomatoes, oregano and basil. Season well and bring to the boil. Reduce the heat to medium-low and cook, uncovered, for 15–20 minutes, stirring occasionally.

Add the steaks to the pan and spoon the tomato mixture over them. Cook for 5–6 minutes until heated through, then remove from the heat. Serve immediately with the rocket salad.

Steak tagliata with roasted vine tomatoes

SERVES 4

EASY ✳

Syns per serving
Extra Easy: Free
Original: Free
Green: 16½ Syns

Preparation time: 10 minutes
Cooking time: under 20 minutes

4 strings of cherry tomatoes on the vine, each with about 8 tomatoes
low calorie cooking spray
salt and freshly ground black pepper
4 x 250g/9oz lean sirloin steaks
1 level tsp Dijon mustard
4 tsp balsamic vinegar
100ml/3½fl oz fat free vinaigrette
75g/3oz wild rocket leaves

Try something different with this quick, delicious and easy sirloin steak dish with roasted vine tomatoes. You can also use lean beef fillet steaks.

Preheat the oven to 180°C/Gas 4. Put the cherry tomatoes into a small roasting tin, spray with low calorie cooking spray and season well. Roast in the oven for 12–15 minutes, until the tomatoes are just tender.

Meanwhile, spray the steaks on both sides with low calorie cooking spray and season to taste. Heat a heavy-based griddle or frying pan over a high heat until smoking. Add the steaks and cook for 2 minutes on each side for rare, 3 minutes for medium and 4 minutes for well-done. Lift onto a board, cover and leave to rest.

Mix the mustard and balsamic vinegar in a small bowl, then whisk in the vinaigrette. Season to taste with salt and pepper.

Serve the steaks with the roasted tomatoes and rocket leaves, drizzled with the balsamic dressing.

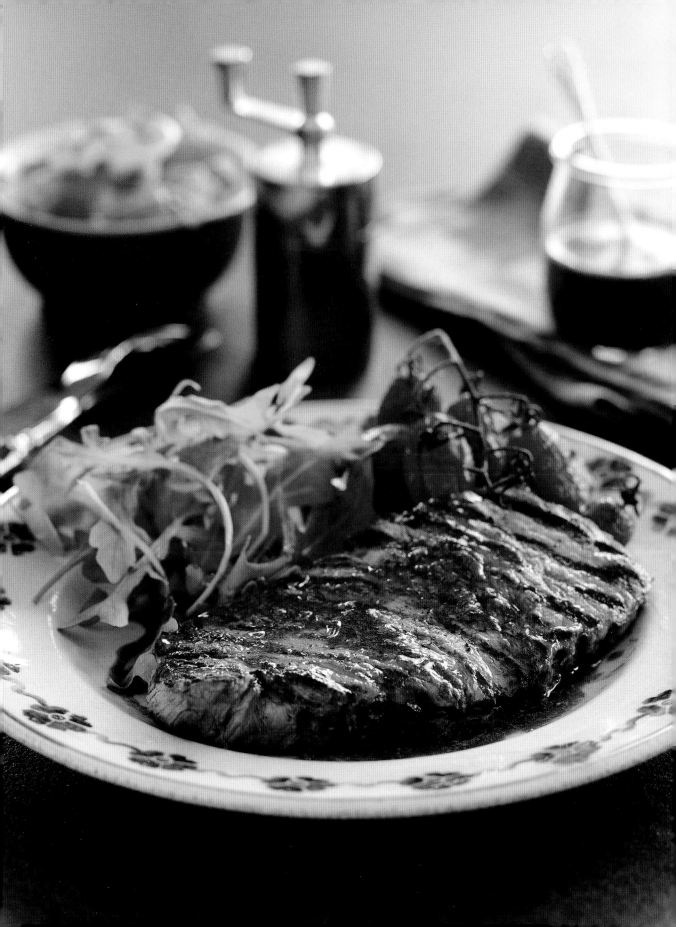

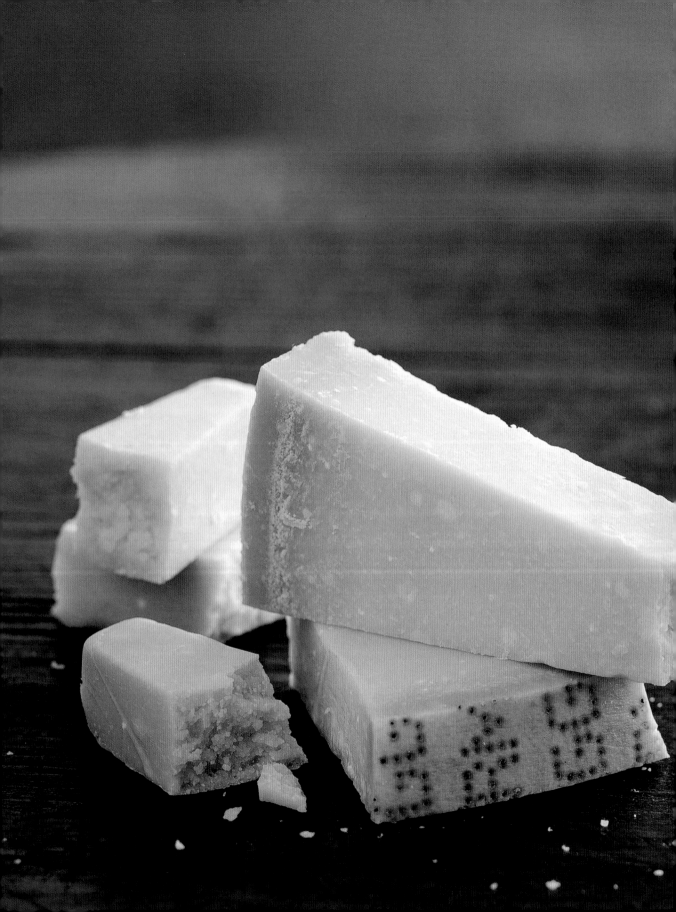

Chapter 6

Vegetarian mains

You will rarely see a plate of plain vegetables on an Italian table; they are often combined into colourful dishes that also make substantial and tasty main courses. Add in a serving of beans or lentils, as in our Tuscan Vegetable and Cannellini Bean Stew (see page 172), and no one will miss the meat. And because many pasta and risotto dishes are made with vegetables, they are perfect as meat-free main meals too. Our choice of vegetable dishes features seasonal ingredients that Italy is famous for, as in Roman Wild Mushroom and Tarragon Bake (see page 157), as well as favourites such as Homemade Tomato Pizza and Melanzane alla Parmigiana (see pages 171 and 163).

Peperonata

SERVES 4

EASY Ⓥ ❄

Syns per serving
Extra Easy: ½ Syn
Original: ½ Syn
Green: ½ Syn

Preparation time: 30 minutes
Cooking time: under 1 hour

2 red peppers
2 green peppers
2 yellow peppers
low calorie cooking spray
2 garlic cloves, peeled and finely
chopped
2 tbsp capers, rinsed
16 black olives, pitted
salt and freshly ground black pepper
4 tbsp chopped parsley
4 tbsp chopped basil
400g can chopped tomatoes
cooked pasta, to serve

This southern Italian dish of stewed peppers in tomato sauce is a firm family favourite in Italy. It makes a great vegetarian main course when served with pasta or it can be served as a side dish with grilled meats and fish.

Preheat the oven to 220°C/Gas 7.

Place the peppers in a roasting tray and roast in the oven for 20 minutes until softened. Transfer to a large bowl, cover with cling film and set aside to cool. Peel the peppers and cut into 5mm/½in thick strips.

Spray a large non-stick frying pan with low calorie cooking spray. Add the garlic and fry gently, over a medium-low heat for 2–3 minutes or until softened.

Add the pepper strips, capers and olives. Season well and cook for 3 minutes.

Add the herbs and tomatoes and cook for a further 25–30 minutes over a low heat, stirring the sauce occasionally.

Remove from the heat and serve immediately with the pasta (1½ Syns per 25g/1oz cooked on Original) of your choice.

Roman wild mushroom and tarragon bake

This tasty vegetable bake is a great family recipe and is the perfect way for getting some vegetables into your kids – and into you too!

SERVES 4

EASY (V) (✱)

Syns per serving
Extra Easy: 5½ Syns
Green: 5½ Syns
Original: 9½ Syns

Preparation time: 20–25 minutes
Cooking time: under 55 minutes

low calorie cooking spray
1 large onion, peeled and
finely chopped
150g/5oz chestnut mushrooms,
thinly sliced
1 red pepper, deseeded and sliced
1 yellow pepper, deseeded and sliced
400g can butter beans,
drained and rinsed
200g/7oz Total 0% Natural
Greek Yogurt
1 garlic clove, peeled and crushed
3 large eggs, beaten
1 tbsp finely chopped tarragon
salt and freshly ground black pepper
225g/8oz reduced fat mozzarella
cheese, cut into cubes

Preheat the oven to 190°C/Gas 5.

Spray a large non-stick frying pan with low calorie cooking spray and place over a high heat. Add the onion, mushrooms and peppers and stir-fry for 6–8 minutes. Remove from the heat, add the beans and transfer this mixture to an ovenproof dish.

In a bowl, whisk together the yogurt, garlic, eggs and tarragon and season well.

Spoon the egg mixture over the vegetables and sprinkle over the cheese. Bake in the oven for 40–45 minutes or until golden and bubbling. Serve immediately.

Napoletana griddled vegetable platter

SERVES 4

EASY

Syns per serving
Extra Easy: 6 Syns
Original: 6 Syns
Green: 6 Syns

Preparation time: 20 minutes
Cooking time: under 20 minutes

6 tbsp balsamic vinegar
2 garlic cloves, peeled and crushed
1 tsp dried basil
1 tsp dried oregano
¼ tsp dried chilli flakes
salt and freshly ground black pepper
1 courgette, cut lengthways
into thin slices
1 medium aubergine,
cut into thin slices
1 red pepper, deseeded and
cut into thin strips
1 yellow pepper, deseeded and
cut into thin strips
50g/2oz wild rocket leaves
110g/4oz Parmesan cheese,
shaved or grated

This vegetarian platter is the perfect thing to serve on a hot summer's day – it can be eaten warm or at room temperature, making it ideal for fuss-free entertaining.

In a large bowl stir together the balsamic vinegar, garlic, basil, oregano and chilli flakes. Season well. Add the vegetables and toss to coat well.

Heat a non-stick griddle over high heat.

Remove the vegetables from the balsamic marinade with a slotted spoon (reserving the remaining marinade) and cook the vegetables, in batches, for 2–3 minutes on each side or until tender.

Arrange the rocket leaves on a platter, top with the griddled vegetables and spoon over the reserved marinade. Sprinkle the Parmesan cheese over the top and serve warm or at room temperature.

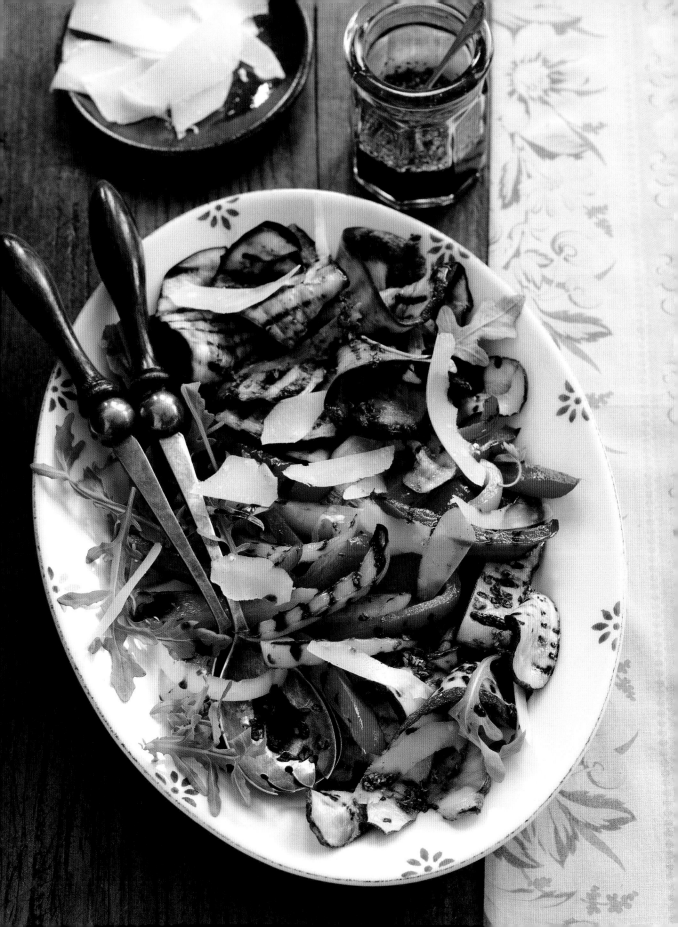

Italian roasted vegetable torta

SERVES 4

WORTH THE EFFORT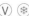

Syns per serving
Extra Easy: 2 Syns
Original: 2 Syns
Green: 2 Syns

Preparation time: 30 minutes
Cooking time: about 1 hour

1 yellow pepper, deseeded and
cut into 1.5cm/½in pieces
1 red pepper, deseeded and
cut into 1.5cm/½in pieces
1 orange pepper, deseeded and
cut into 1.5cm/½in pieces
2 medium courgettes,
cut into 1.5cm/½in pieces
1 medium aubergine,
cut into 1.5cm/½in pieces
400g can artichoke hearts in water,
drained and halved
1 large onion, peeled and sliced
4 bay leaves
2 rosemary sprigs
2 oregano sprigs
low calorie cooking spray
110g/4oz ricotta cheese, crumbled
4 large eggs, beaten
3 tsp dried Italian mixed herbs
salt and freshly ground black pepper

This colourful and delicious torta is a treat for vegetarians and meat-eaters alike. It can be made in individual flan dishes, if you prefer.

Preheat the oven to 200°C/Gas 6.

Place the vegetables and fresh herbs in a non-stick roasting tray and spray them with low calorie cooking spray. Bake the vegetables in the oven for 12–15 minutes.

Remove from the oven, discard the bay leaves, rosemary and oregano sprigs and transfer to a large mixing bowl.

When the vegetables are cool, mix in the ricotta cheese, eggs and dried herbs. Season well.

Pack the mixture into a 25cm/10in diameter ovenproof flan dish, place in the oven and bake for 30–40 minutes or until the mixture is set and golden.

Serve warm or at room temperature.

Stuffed cabbage leaves

This slow-cooked dish of cabbage leaves stuffed with leek, mushrooms and rice is perfect for when the weather turns cool and you need delicious comfort food.

SERVES 4

WORTH THE EFFORT Ⓥ

Syns per serving
Extra Easy: Free
Green: Free
Original: 7½ Syns

Preparation time: 30 minutes
Cooking time: about 1¼ hours

12 large Savoy cabbage leaves
low calorie cooking spray
1 leek, trimmed and finely chopped
200g/7oz mushrooms, finely chopped
2 tsp finely chopped rosemary
1 celery stick, finely chopped
175g/6oz dried long grain rice
salt and freshly ground black pepper
400ml/14fl oz vegetable stock
1 tbsp balsamic vinegar

Preheat the oven to 160°C/Gas 3.

Remove the tough central stalk from each of the cabbage leaves. Bring a large pan of salted water to the boil, add the cabbage and cook for just 1–2 minutes or until the leaves are starting to wilt. Drain and refresh under cold running water. Drain well and pat dry with kitchen paper.

Spray a non-stick frying pan with low calorie cooking spray and place over a medium heat. Add the leek and mushrooms and fry for 10 minutes or until lightly browned. Add the rosemary and celery and cook for a further 5–6 minutes.

Stir in the rice and cook for a minute or so until the grains are glistening. Remove from the heat and season well.

Spoon a little stuffing onto a cabbage leaf, roll up and fold in the sides to enclose the filling. Fill the remaining leaves in the same way.

Place in a large and shallow ovenproof dish in a single layer with the join underneath. Mix together the stock and vinegar and pour over the cabbage.

Cover the dish tightly with foil and bake for 1 hour. Uncover and cook for a further 15 minutes. Serve warm or at room temperature.

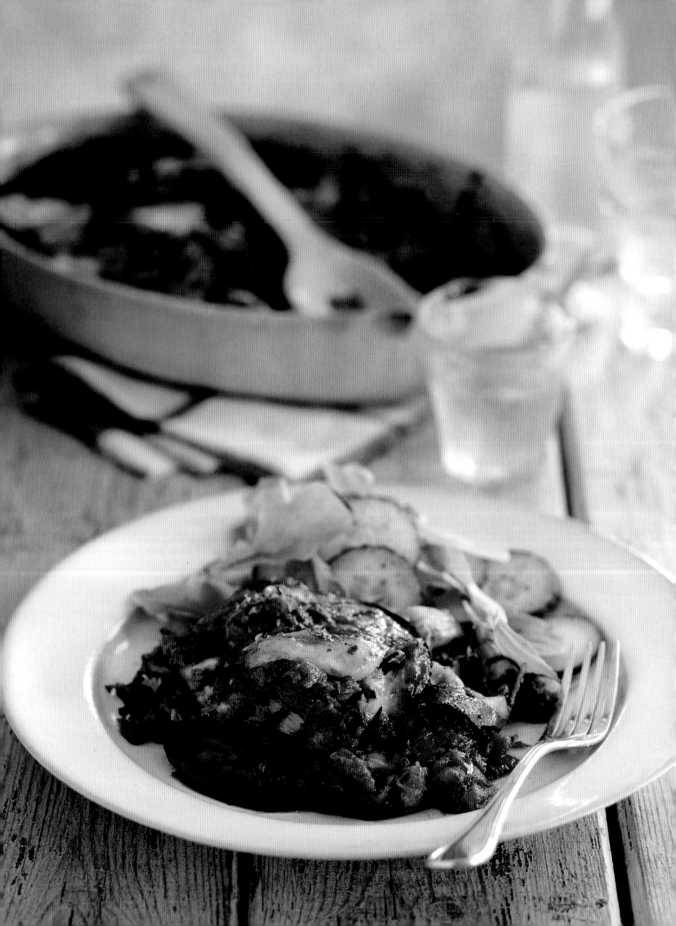

Melanzane alla parmigiana

In this southern Italian dish, the aubergines are first cooked on a griddle to add more flavour before being baked with a wonderfully colourful tomato and cheese sauce.

SERVES 4

WORTH THE EFFORT

Syns per serving
Extra Easy: 5½ Syns
Original: 5½ Syns
Green: 5½ Syns

Preparation time: 25–30 minutes
Cooking time: about 1 hour

low calorie cooking spray
4 garlic cloves, peeled and thinly sliced
2 x 400g cans chopped tomatoes
2 tsp dried basil
2 tsp dried oregano
½ tsp dried chilli flakes
¼ tsp artificial sweetener
40g/1½oz basil leaves, finely shredded
salt and freshly ground black pepper
3 medium aubergines
225g/8oz reduced fat mozzarella cheese, sliced
chopped parsley, to serve

Preheat the oven to 160°C/Gas 3.

Spray a large non-stick frying pan with low calorie cooking spray, add the garlic and stir-fry over a medium heat for 1–2 minutes.

Add the tomatoes, dried basil, oregano, chilli flakes and sweetener and simmer for 15 minutes until thickened. Stir in the basil leaves and season well.

Meanwhile, cut the aubergines lengthways into 5mm/½in thick slices. Spray both sides with low calorie cooking spray, season and cook in batches on a non-stick griddle or non-stick frying pan, for 2–3 minutes on each side or until tender.

Place a few spoonfuls of the tomato sauce in the bottom of a medium ovenproof dish. Cover with the aubergine and mozzarella slices then repeat, ending with a layer of mozzarella (you'll have roughly 5–7 layers).

Place in the oven and bake for 25–30 minutes until golden and bubbling. Remove from the oven and serve garnished with chopped parsley.

Timballo of rice, leek and courgette

SERVES 4

WORTH THE EFFORT ❋

Syns per serving
Extra Easy: 6 Syns
Green: 6 Syns
Original: 17½ Syns

Preparation time: 20–25 minutes
Cooking time: about 1¼ hour s

low calorie cooking spray
1 onion, peeled and finely chopped
2 garlic cloves, peeled and crushed
250g/9oz dried risotto rice
1 tbsp chopped thyme
850ml/1½ pints vegetable stock
a large pinch of saffron threads
110g/4oz Parmesan cheese, grated
1 leek, trimmed and thinly sliced
200g/7oz baby courgettes, thinly sliced
a pinch of nutmeg
salt and freshly ground black pepper

Timballo is the Italian word for large kettle drum. This rice and vegetable mould makes an impressive main course for a special occasion.

Spray a large non-stick saucepan with low calorie cooking spray and cook the onion and garlic for 5–6 minutes over a low heat. Add the rice and thyme and stir until well coated.

Bring the stock and saffron to the boil, then reduce the heat to a simmer. Stir in the stock a ladleful at a time, stirring constantly, until it is absorbed. Repeat this step until the rice is cooked. (This will take 25–30 minutes.) Remove from the heat and stir in the Parmesan cheese.

Spray a non-stick frying pan with low calorie cooking spray, add the leek and stir-fry for 4–5 minutes over a high heat. Add the courgette and cook for 5 minutes. Add the nutmeg and season.

Preheat the oven to 180°C/Gas 4. Spray a 1.5 litre/ 2½ pint pudding basin with low calorie cooking spray and line the base with baking parchment.

Put half of the rice mixture into the pudding basin, pressing it down firmly, and then spoon over the leek and courgette mixture. Add the remaining rice, again pressing down firmly. Cover with foil and bake in the oven for 20–25 minutes. Allow to rest for 10 minutes. Run a palette knife around the edge of the bowl before turning out onto a serving platter. Serve immediately.

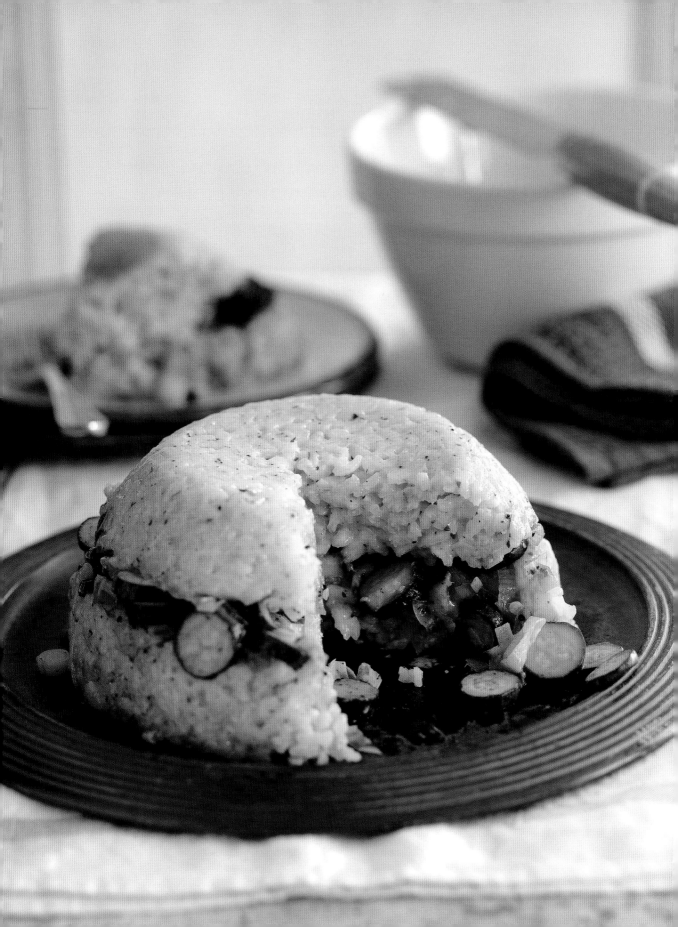

Roasted peppers stuffed with pasta, cherry tomatoes and herbs

SERVES 4

WORTH THE EFFORT ✳

Syns per serving
Extra Easy: 5½ Syns
Green: 5½ Syns
Original: 8 Syns

Preparation time: 25 minutes
Cooking time: 20–25 minutes

4 large red peppers
50g/2oz very thin dried spaghetti
12 cherry tomatoes, quartered
3 garlic cloves, peeled and crushed
4 tbsp finely chopped basil
110g/4oz Pecorino cheese, grated
salt and freshly ground black pepper

This dish is a vegetable and pasta course in one. The garlic-flavoured tomatoes keep the pasta moist.

Preheat the oven to 220°C/Gas 7.

Slice the tops off the peppers and reserve. Scoop out the seeds with a small spoon and discard. Place the peppers upright in an ovenproof dish that is small enough to fit them snugly.

Cook the pasta according to the packet instructions.

Place the tomatoes in a bowl with the garlic, basil and Pecorino cheese. Season well with salt and pepper and mix thoroughly.

Fill the peppers two-thirds full with the pasta and then top with the tomato mixture. Place the pepper lids on top, stand them in a roasting tin and bake in the oven for 20–25 minutes or until the peppers start to soften.

Serve warm or at room temperature.

Potato and mushroom gratin

SERVES 4

EASY ❋

Syns per serving
Extra Easy: 6 Syns
Green: 6 Syns
Original: 15½ Syns

Preparation time: 30 minutes
Cooking time: 1 hour and 10 minutes

1kg/2lb 4oz medium-sized potatoes
(Desiree or Maris Piper), peeled and
very thinly sliced
750g/1lb 10oz large flat mushrooms,
thickly sliced
110g/4oz Parmesan cheese, grated
8 tbsp finely chopped flat-leaf parsley
salt and freshly ground black pepper
a crisp green salad, to serve

Baking the mushrooms and potatoes in layers allows the potato to absorb the mushroom juices in this delicious one-pot recipe.

Preheat the oven to 180°C/Gas 4.

Place half of the potato slices in the base of an ovenproof dish and cover with half of the mushroom slices.

Mix together the Parmesan and parsley in a bowl and season well. Spread half the mixture over the mushrooms, cover with the remaining potatoes and mushrooms and then top with the rest of the herby cheese.

Cover with foil and bake in the oven for 1 hour, then remove the foil and bake for a further 10 minutes, or until the potatoes are tender.

Serve immediately with the green salad.

Southern Italian torta

SERVES 4

EASY Ⓥ ❋

This potato, cheese and herb cake is delicious to eat and makes an impressive centrepiece for a summer lunch or picnic.

Syns per serving
Extra Easy: 2½ Syns
Green: 2½ Syns
Original: 14 Syns

Preparation time: 30–40 minutes
Cooking time: just over 1 hour

1.2kg/2lb 10oz floury potatoes (Maris Piper or King Edward)
300g/11oz fat free natural fromage frais
4 eggs, lightly beaten
2 garlic cloves, peeled and crushed
2 tbsp finely chopped thyme
6 tbsp finely chopped flat-leaf parsley
110g/4oz reduced fat mozzarella cheese, finely diced
1 tsp dried chilli flakes
salt and freshly ground black pepper
low calorie cooking spray
chopped thyme, to garnish
Treviso leaves, to serve (aka Italian red salad leaves)

Preheat the oven to 160°C/Gas 3.

Boil the potatoes whole, in their skins, in gently simmering water for 30–40 minutes, depending on their size, until tender. Drain the potatoes thoroughly.

When cool enough to handle, peel the potatoes, cut into big chunks, then tip back into the pan. Add the fromage frais and mash until fairly smooth. Mix in the eggs, garlic, herbs, mozzarella cheese and chilli flakes and season well.

Lightly spray the inside of a 23cm/9in spring-form tin with low calorie cooking spray and spoon in the potato mixture. Smooth down the surface.

Bake for about 1 hour or until the potato cake is set, with a slight wobble in the middle.

Let the torta rest for 5 minutes, then carefully loosen from the sides with a knife before releasing it from the tin. Slide onto a plate and garnish with the thyme leaves. Serve hot or warm with the Treviso leaves.

Tip This recipe can be prepared up to the end of step 4 the night before and kept covered in the fridge until ready to bake.

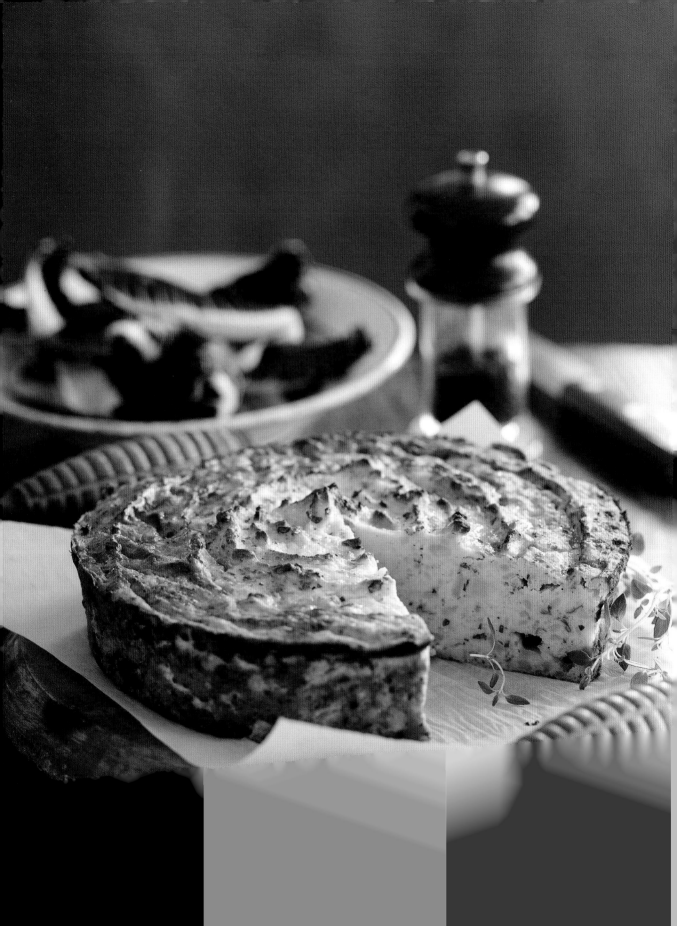

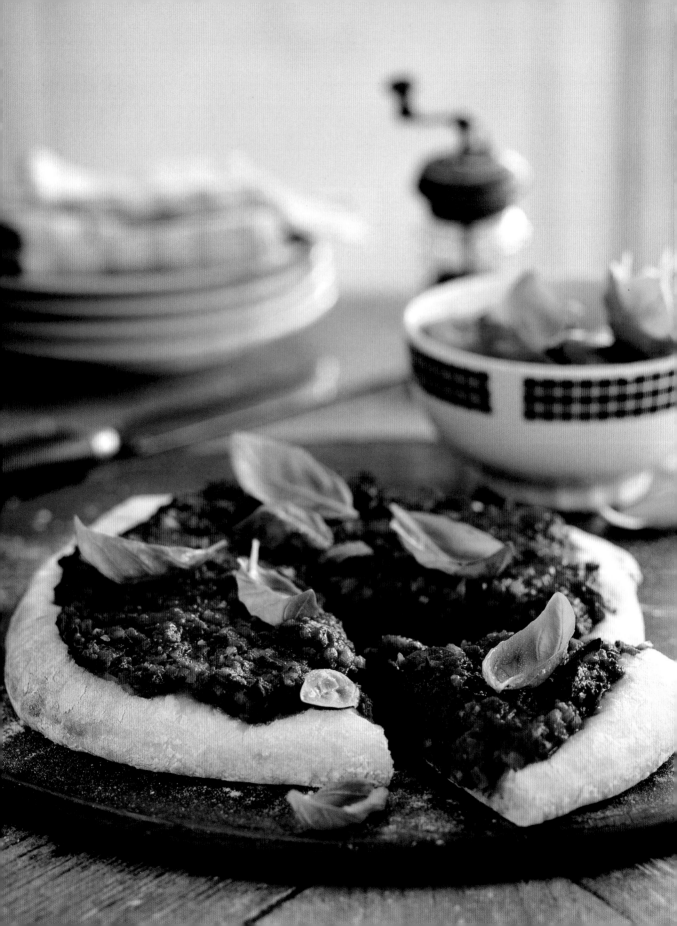

Homemade tomato pizza

MAKES ONE PIZZA (SERVES 6–8)

WORTH THE EFFORT

Syns per serving (serves 6)
Extra Easy: 4½ Syns
Original: 4½ Syns
Green: 4½ Syns

Syns per serving (serves 8)
Extra Easy: 3½ Syns
Original: 3½ Syns
Green: 3½ Syns

Preparation time: about 1 hour
Cooking time: 12–15 minutes

FOR THE PIZZA BASE
145g sachet dried pizza base mix

FOR THE TOPPING
4 shallots, peeled and finely chopped
3 cloves of garlic, peeled and crushed
2 tsp dried oregano
2 tbsp finely chopped basil
400g can chopped tomatoes
1 level tbsp sun-dried tomato purée
salt and freshly ground black pepper

This recipe makes a basic tomato-topped pizza. Feel free to add any other toppings you like, such as basil, vegetables, rocket, red onion and mozzarella, and amend the Syns accordingly.

Make up the pizza base according to the packet instructions.

Meanwhile, put the shallots, garlic, oregano, basil, tomatoes and tomato purée into a saucepan and cook over a medium-low heat for 25–30 minutes or until you have a thick spreadable sauce. Season well.

Preheat the oven to 220°C/Gas 7.

Turn the pizza dough out onto a well floured surface. Form the dough into a round ball and roll out into a pizza base shape. Spread the tomato sauce over the base and bake in the oven for 12–15 minutes or until golden brown.

Tuscan vegetable and cannellini bean stew

SERVES 4

EASY (V) (❋)

Syns per serving
Extra Easy: Free
Green: Free
Original: 8½ Syns

Preparation time: 20 minutes
Cooking time: under 1 hour

low calorie cooking spray
2 red onions, peeled and thinly sliced
4 garlic cloves, peeled and crushed
1 tsp chilli powder (optional)
2 carrots, peeled and sliced
4 celery sticks, sliced
4 plum tomatoes, peeled, deseeded
and roughly chopped
2 thyme sprigs
2 bay leaves
salt and freshly ground black pepper
350ml/12fl oz vegetable stock
2 x 400g cans cannellini beans,
drained and rinsed
100g/3½oz green beans, trimmed and
cut into short lengths

This warming and wholesome dish is kept fresh and light with the addition of the tomatoes and green beans. Serve it with rice or a crisp green salad.

Spray a non-stick frying pan with low calorie cooking spray, add the onions and cook over a medium-low heat for 10 minutes or until softened.

Add the garlic and chilli powder, if using, and stir-fry for 1–2 minutes. Then add the carrots, celery, tomatoes, thyme sprigs and bay leaves and season well.

Pour in the stock, bring to the boil and simmer, stirring occasionally, for 20–30 minutes or until the vegetables are tender.

Add all the beans, then simmer for 5–10 minutes or until the cannellini beans have heated through and the green beans are just tender. Serve hot.

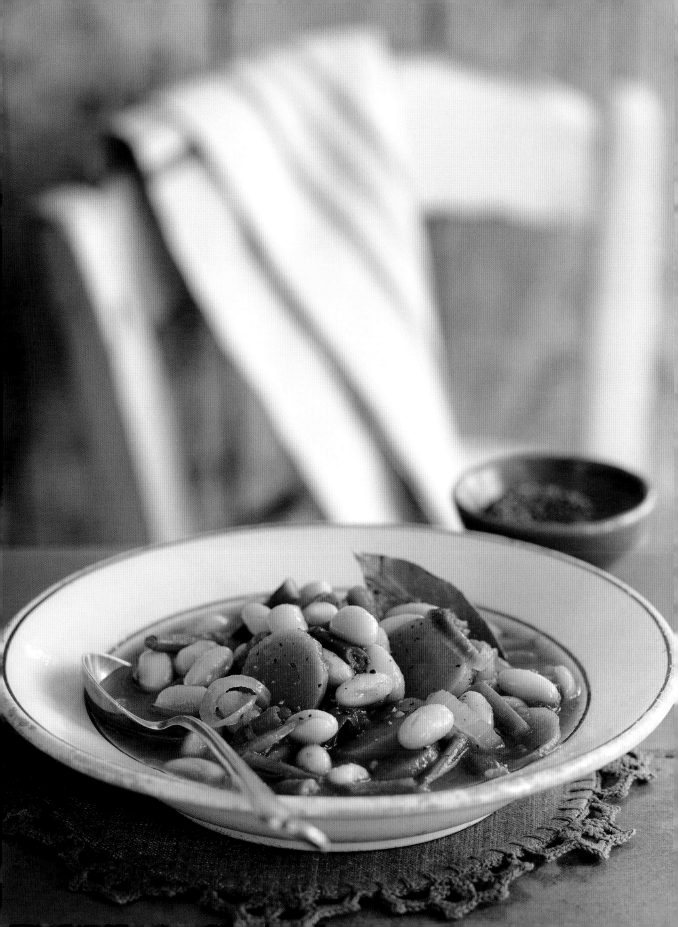

Cannelloni

SERVES 4

WORTH THE EFFORT (V) (✳)

Syns per serving
Extra Easy: 2 Syns
Green: 2 Syns
Original: 7½ Syns

Preparation time: 20 minutes
Cooking time: 25 minutes

400g/14oz quark
110g/4oz ricotta cheese
1 small egg, lightly beaten
75g/3oz wild rocket leaves, finely chopped
2 tbsp finely chopped basil
4 garlic cloves, peeled and crushed
¼ tsp grated nutmeg
salt and freshly ground black pepper
6 dried lasagne sheets, cooked
400g can cherry tomatoes
300g/11oz passata with garlic and herbs
a crisp green salad, to serve

This cannelloni recipe combines creamy Italian ricotta cheese, speckled with slightly bitter rocket and a rich tomato sauce. The contrast between the sauce and the filling is terrific.

Preheat the oven to 200°C/Gas 6.

Place the quark and ricotta cheese in a bowl and break it up with a fork. Add the egg, rocket, basil, garlic and nutmeg and season well. Mix until well combined.

Cut each lasagne sheet into half. Spread 2–3 tablespoons of the ricotta mixture down the centre of each sheet and then roll into a tube, overlapping the edges slightly.

Mix together the canned cherry tomatoes and passata and season.

Spread a layer of the tomato mixture over the base of an 18 x 25cm/7 x 10in ovenproof dish.

Place the filled cannelloni tubes, seam side down, in a single layer in the dish and pour over the remaining tomato mixture. Bake in the oven for 20–25 minutes or until bubbling.

Remove from the oven and serve with a crisp green salad.

Italian Quorn sausage and borlotti bean stew

SERVES 4

EASY (V)

Syns per serving
Extra Easy: Free
Green: Free
Original: 5 Syns

Preparation time: 25–30 minutes
Cooking time: just over 1 hour

low calorie cooking spray
8 plain Quorn sausages, cut into
bite-sized chunks
1 onion, peeled and chopped
2 garlic cloves, peeled and
finely chopped
3 carrots, peeled and finely chopped
3 celery sticks, finely chopped
1 leek, trimmed and finely chopped
400ml/14fl oz vegetable stock
1 bay leaf
salt and freshly ground black pepper
400g can borlotti beans,
drained and rinsed
chopped parsley, to garnish

This comforting, hearty stew comes from Emilia-Romagna, the gastronomic centre of Italy.

Spray a large, deep non-stick pan with low calorie cooking spray and place over a medium heat. Add the sausages, onion, garlic, carrots, celery and leek, stir well and cook for 10–12 minutes until the onion begins to soften.

Stir in the stock and bay leaf and season well with salt and pepper. Bring to the boil, reduce the heat to medium-low and simmer for 40 minutes or until the sausages are cooked through and the vegetables are tender.

Add the borlotti beans 10 minutes before the end of the cooking time. Remove from the heat and garnish with chopped parsley before serving.

Wild mixed mushroom lasagne

SERVES 4

EASY Ⓥ ✳

Syns per serving
Extra Easy: 5½ Syns
Green: 5½ Syns
Original: 12½ Syns

Preparation time: 30 minutes
Cooking time: around 1 hour

low calorie cooking spray
2 garlic cloves, peeled and crushed
300g/11oz mixed mushrooms,
roughly chopped
1 onion, peeled and finely chopped
1 fennel bulb, trimmed and
finely chopped
2 x 400g cans chopped tomatoes
100ml/3½fl oz vegetable stock
salt and freshly ground black pepper
8 dried lasagne sheets
225g/8oz reduced fat
mozzarella cheese
chopped basil, to serve
mixed salad leaves, to serve

Use any combination of mushrooms for this delicious lasagne – just make sure that they're fresh and firm. Chestnut, porcini, button and large field mushrooms are particularly good as they are quite meaty in texture.

Preheat the oven to 180°C/Gas 4.

Spray a large heavy-based pan with low calorie cooking spray and place over a medium heat. Add the garlic, mushrooms, onion and fennel and cook for 6–8 minutes until softened.

Add the tomatoes and stock, season well and bring to the boil. Simmer gently for 20–25 minutes until the vegetables are cooked through and tender.

To assemble the lasagne, spoon one-third of the tomato and mushroom sauce into the base of a lasagne dish. Add a layer of lasagne sheets and then spoon over another layer of the sauce.

Break the mozzarella into rough pieces and scatter a third of it evenly over the sauce.

Continue to layer up the dish until all the ingredients are used up, finishing with a layer of the remaining cheese.

Bake in the oven for 25–30 minutes until golden and bubbling, garnish with chopped basil and serve immediately with mixed salad leaves.

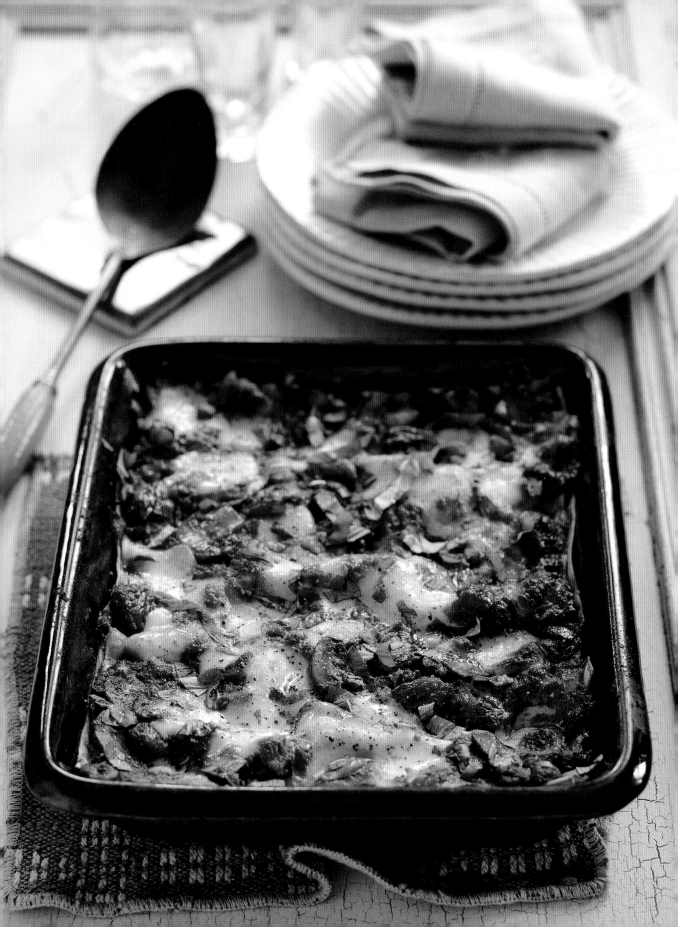

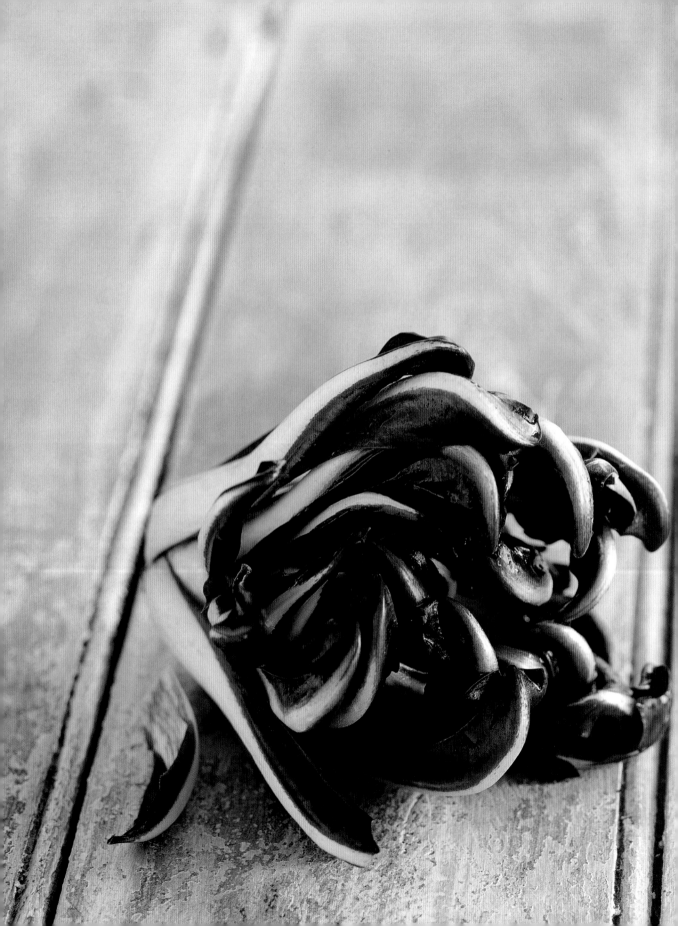

Chapter 7

Sides and accompaniments

Accompaniments and side dishes are never an afterthought in Italy, and it's no surprise when classic recipes include Slow Roasted Plum Tomatoes with Oregano and Garlic, Sautéed Spinach with Raisins, and Rosemary Roasties (see pages 180, 195 and 196). Often, side dishes include meat or beans as well as vegetables, giving even more variety in texture and flavour – for example, when fresh peas are transformed with slivers of prosciutto (ham), or butternut squash is sautéed and mixed with crispy pancetta (bacon) and thyme. Getting the family to eat up their greens (and yellows, reds and oranges) has never been easier.

Slow roasted plum tomatoes with oregano and garlic

SERVES 4

EASY Ⓥ

Syns per serving
Extra Easy: Free
Original: Free
Green: Free

Preparation time: 10 minutes
Cooking time: 1½ hours

10 plum tomatoes, halved lengthways
2 garlic cloves, peeled and finely chopped
1 tbsp dried oregano
sea salt and freshly ground black pepper
low calorie cooking spray

Tomatoes cooked with oregano and garlic just burst with the flavours of the Mediterranean. Use the ripest plum tomatoes you can for maximum flavour.

Preheat the oven to 140°C/Gas 1 and line a baking tray with non-stick baking parchment.

Place the tomatoes, cut side up, on the baking tray. Sprinkle over the garlic and oregano and season well. Spray with low calorie cooking spray and cook in the oven for 1½ hours or until the tomatoes have shrunk and have turned deep red in colour.

Remove from the oven and serve warm or at room temperature.

Griddled aubergine with mint

SERVES 4

EASY (V)

Syns per serving
Extra Easy: Free
Original: Free
Green: Free

Preparation time: 10 minutes
Cooking time: about 10–15 minutes

2 large aubergines, ends trimmed and cut into 5mm/¼in thick slices
1 fresh red chilli, deseeded and finely chopped
salt and freshly ground black pepper
low calorie cooking spray
juice of 1 lemon
4–5 tbsp aged balsamic vinegar
a large handful of finely chopped mint

In Italy this dish is served as an accompaniment to grilled lamb, but you could also serve it as a starter with wild rocket.

Toss the aubergine slices in a bowl with the red chilli and season well.

Heat a non-stick ridged griddle until hot. Spray the aubergine slices with low calorie cooking spray and cook the slices in batches for about 2 minutes on each side, until they are tender but still retaining a slight crunch to them. Drain on kitchen paper.

Place the aubergine slices in a shallow bowl in a single layer. Drizzle over the lemon juice and balsamic vinegar and scatter over the mint.

Serve warm or at room temperature.

Artichoke hearts with a lemon and mint dressing

SERVES 4

WORTH THE EFFORT Ⓥ

Syns per serving
Extra Easy: Free
Original: Free
Green: Free

Preparation time: 30 minutes
Cooking time: under 45 minutes

4 large, fresh artichokes
3 bay leaves
1 lemon, cut in half
1 tsp finely chopped red pepper,
to serve
mint leaves, to serve

FOR THE MINT DRESSING
a large handful of mint, finely chopped
2 garlic cloves, peeled and crushed
juice of 2 lemons
100ml/3½fl oz fat free vinaigrette
salt and freshly ground black pepper

Artichokes grow all over Italy, but Rome is renowned for its very young and tender variety. Buy the freshest artichokes you can find for this recipe.

Prepare the artichokes by trimming the base of the stalk and then peel the stem with a sharp knife. Cut off 10mm from the top of the artichoke.

Place the bay leaves, lemon halves and artichokes in a large saucepan (the artichokes should fit snugly) and pour over enough cold water to cover. Bring to the boil, cover, reduce the heat and simmer for 35–40 minutes until the artichokes are softened. Remove them from the pan and drain. Remove all the leaves from the artichokes and scoop out the central 'choke' with a teaspoon.

To make the dressing, mix together all the ingredients in a bowl and season well.

Halve the artichokes lengthways and pour over the dressing. Serve warm or at room temperature garnished with the red pepper and mint leaves.

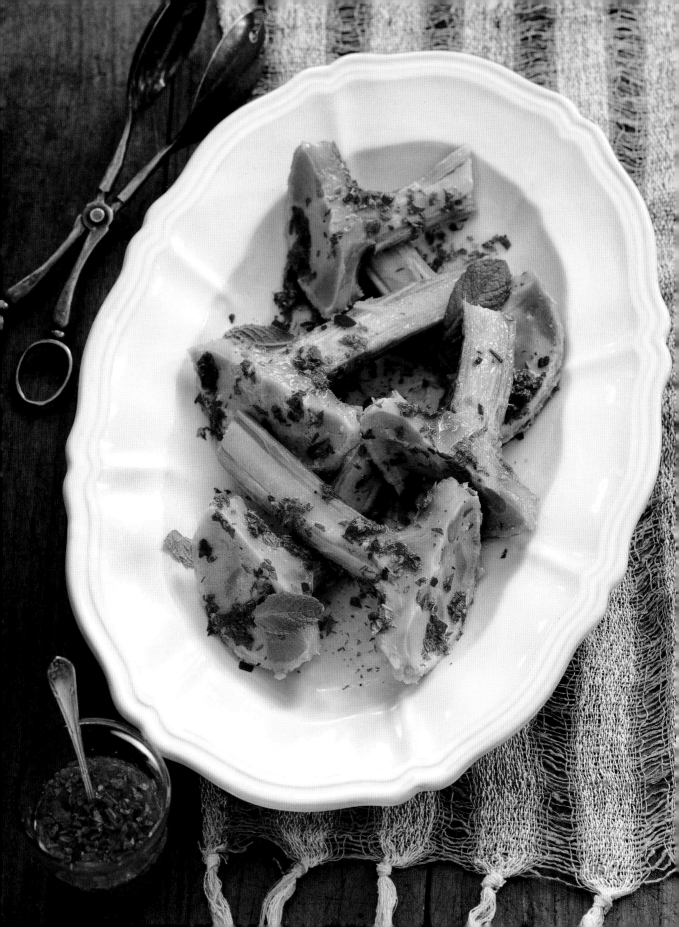

Fresh peas with prosciutto

In this recipe, fresh peas are cooked very quickly with sautéed spring onions and chopped salty Italian prosciutto. You can use lean bacon instead of the prosciutto, and frozen peas if fresh peas are not in season.

SERVES 4

REALLY EASY ✳

Syns per serving
Extra Easy: 1 Syn
Green: 2½ Syns
Original: 6 Syns

Preparation time: 10 minutes
Cooking time: under 15 minutes

low calorie cooking spray
2 bunches of spring onions, trimmed and roughly sliced
6 slices of prosciutto, roughly chopped
500g/1lb 2oz fresh peas, shelled
125ml/4½fl oz boiling hot vegetable stock
a small handful of flat-leaf parsley, finely chopped

Spray a large non-stick frying pan with low calorie cooking spray and place over a medium heat.

Add the spring onions and prosciutto and sauté for 5–6 minutes or until the onions are translucent.

Add the peas and the vegetable stock. Bring to a simmer and cook, uncovered, for 6–8 minutes or until the peas are tender (if using frozen peas cook for 2–3 minutes).

Drain the peas and toss with the chopped parsley. Serve warm.

Broccoli with chilli and garlic

SERVES 4

EASY Ⓥ ❋

Syns per serving
Extra Easy: Free
Original: Free
Green: Free

Preparation time: 10 minutes
Cooking time: under 10 minutes

650g/1lb 7oz broccoli,
cut into small florets
salt
low calorie cooking spray
2 garlic cloves, peeled and finely sliced
1 mild red chilli, deseeded and
thinly sliced

This recipe is the simple classic way of cooking broccoli in Italy. To turn it into a main course, simply toss with cooked spaghetti or linguine. If you like your food hot, you can leave the seeds in the chillies.

Cook the broccoli in a large saucepan of lightly salted boiling water for 3–4 minutes or until just tender. Drain well.

Spray a large non-stick frying pan with low calorie cooking spray and place over a low heat. Add the garlic and chilli and stir-fry for 1–2 minutes.

Increase the heat to high, add the broccoli and stir-fry for 1–2 minutes.

Serve immediately.

Char-grilled radicchio

SERVES 4

EASY Ⓥ

Syns per serving
Extra Easy: 1½ Syns
Original: 1½ Syns
Green: 1½ Syns

Preparation time: 5 minutes
Cooking time: under 10 minutes

2 round radicchios, cut into quarters
low calorie cooking spray
salt and freshly ground black pepper
4 level tbsp grated Parmesan cheese

Radicchio is a member of the chicory family and its bitter peppery taste makes it a perfect accompaniment to many grilled chicken, meat and fish dishes.

Preheat the grill to medium-high.

Lightly spray the radicchio quarters with low calorie cooking spray and season well.

Place the quarters, cut side up, on a baking sheet and cook under the grill, about 14cm/5½in away from the heat source, for 6–8 minutes. The leaves will darken in colour but they should not start to blacken and burn.

Scatter over the Parmesan cheese and return to the grill for 20–30 seconds or until the cheese just starts to melt.

Serve immediately.

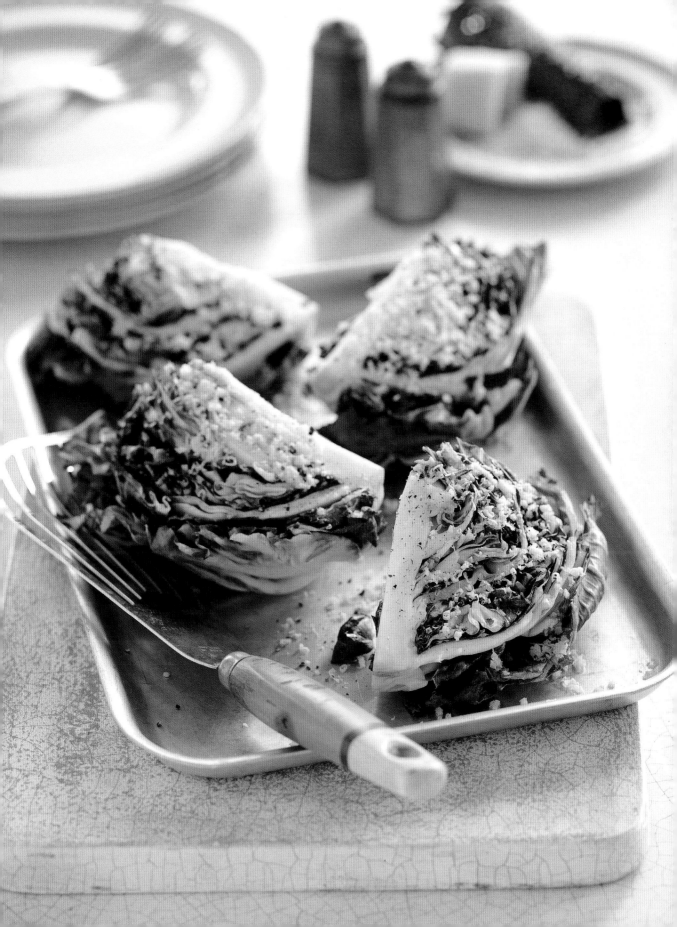

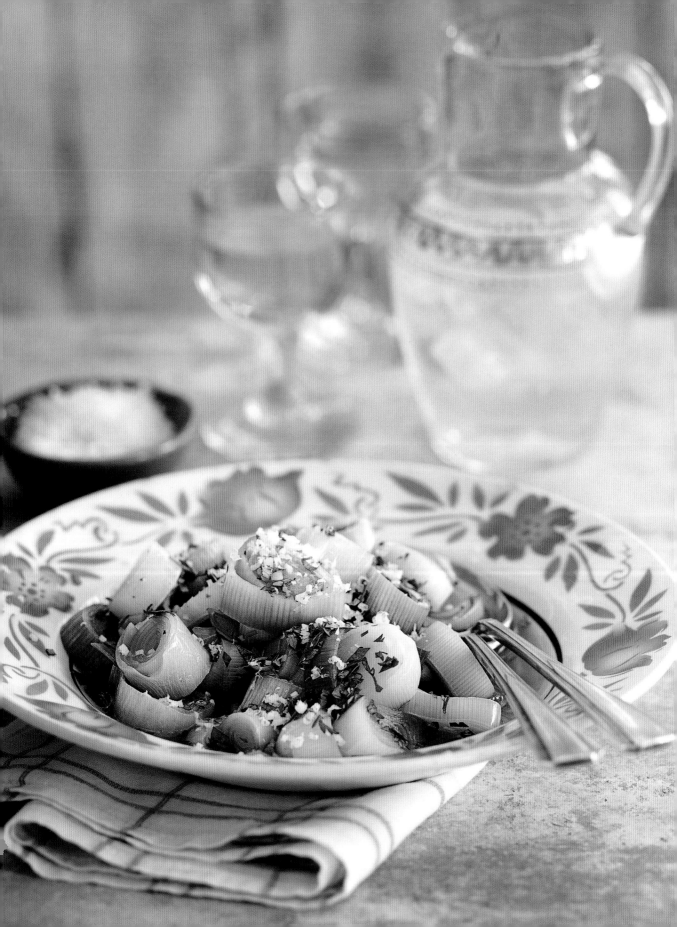

Braised leeks with white wine and herbs

SERVES 4

EASY Ⓥ ❋

Syns per serving
Extra Easy: 1 Syn
Original: 1 Syn
Green: 1 Syn

Preparation time: 10 minutes
Cooking time: under 30 minutes

3 leeks, trimmed and thinly sliced
300ml/11fl oz vegetable stock
100ml/3½fl oz white wine
salt and freshly ground black pepper
2 tbsp finely chopped flat-leaf parsley,
to garnish
grated Parmesan cheese,
to garnish (optional)

When cooked this way the leeks take on a very sweet flavour that is absolutely delicious.

Place the leeks in a saucepan together with the stock and wine.

Bring to the boil, reduce the heat to low, cover and simmer gently for about 20 minutes, stirring occasionally until the leeks are very tender.

Remove from the heat, season well and serve garnished with the parsley and Parmesan cheese, (1½ Syns per level tbsp), if using.

Fennel with garlic and white wine

SERVES 4

EASY (V) (❄)

Syns per serving
Extra Easy: 1½ Syns
Original: 1½ Syns
Green: 1½ Syns

Preparation time: 15 minutes
Cooking time: about 30 minutes

low calorie cooking spray
2 large fennel bulbs, trimmed and cut
into quarters
6–8 large garlic cloves, unpeeled
1 tsp dried red chilli flakes
1 tbsp finely chopped rosemary
125ml/4½fl oz dry white wine
juice of 2 oranges

Fennel is delicious eaten raw in salads but it undergoes a complete transformation when it's cooked; from the fresh aniseed flavour and crisp texture to a robust-tasting vegetable that is tender with a juicy bite. It is fabulous served with grilled fish.

Spray a heavy-based saucepan with low calorie cooking spray. Place the fennel in the saucepan with the garlic, chilli flakes and rosemary. Cook over a medium heat for 10 minutes, stirring occasionally, until lightly golden.

Add the wine and bring to the boil over a high heat, then reduce the heat to medium-low and cook uncovered for 12–15 minutes or until the vegetables are just tender.

Stir in the orange juice and cook for 6–8 minutes.

Season well and serve warm or at room temperature.

Roasted balsamic onions

SERVES 4

EASY Ⓥ ⊛

Syns per serving
Extra Easy: Free
Original: Free
Green: Free

Preparation time: 15 minutes
Cooking time: about 1 hour 10 minutes

4 large red onions
low calorie cooking spray
salt and freshly ground black pepper
4 tbsp aged balsamic vinegar
2 tsp fennel seeds
2 tbsp capers, rinsed
3 tbsp finely chopped flat-leaf parsley

In Sicily onions are baked whole and then squeezed out of their skins after roasting. Here they're flavoured with fennel seeds, capers and balsamic vinegar.

Preheat the oven to 190°C/Gas 5.

Trim the root end of the onions so they can stand up securely. Cut a deep cross in the top of each one, slicing towards the base, almost cutting them into quarters but with the base still intact.

Pack them closely together in an ovenproof dish to fit snugly and spray with low calorie cooking spray. Season well and place in the oven for 1 hour or until tender.

Remove from the oven and drizzle over the balsamic vinegar and fennel seeds and return to the oven for 10 minutes.

To serve, carefully place the onions with all the pan juices onto a dish and scatter over the capers and parsley. Your guests can squeeze the onions out of their skins.

Roasted butternut squash with red peppers

SERVES 4

EASY

Syns per serving
Extra Easy: Free
Original: Free
Green: Free

Preparation time: 15 minutes
Cooking time: 15–20 minutes

1 butternut squash, peeled, deseeded and cut into 2cm/¾in dice
2 red peppers, deseeded and cut into bite-sized pieces
1 garlic clove, peeled and finely chopped
4 thyme sprigs, plus extra to serve
salt and freshly ground black pepper
low calorie cooking spray

This simple and delicious roasted vegetable dish is perfect for the autumnal months when there are lots of different kinds of squash about. You can use any squash you like, but the butternut variety works particularly well. For a non-vegetarian version, add chopped lean bacon or pancetta to the vegetables in the pan before cooking.

Preheat the oven to 200°C/Gas 6.

Put the squash and peppers into a large roasting tray. Sprinkle over the garlic and add the thyme sprigs. Season well and lightly spray with low calorie cooking spray.

Place in the oven to roast for 15–20 minutes or until the vegetables are just tender.

Remove from the oven and serve warm or at room temperature garnished with thyme sprigs.

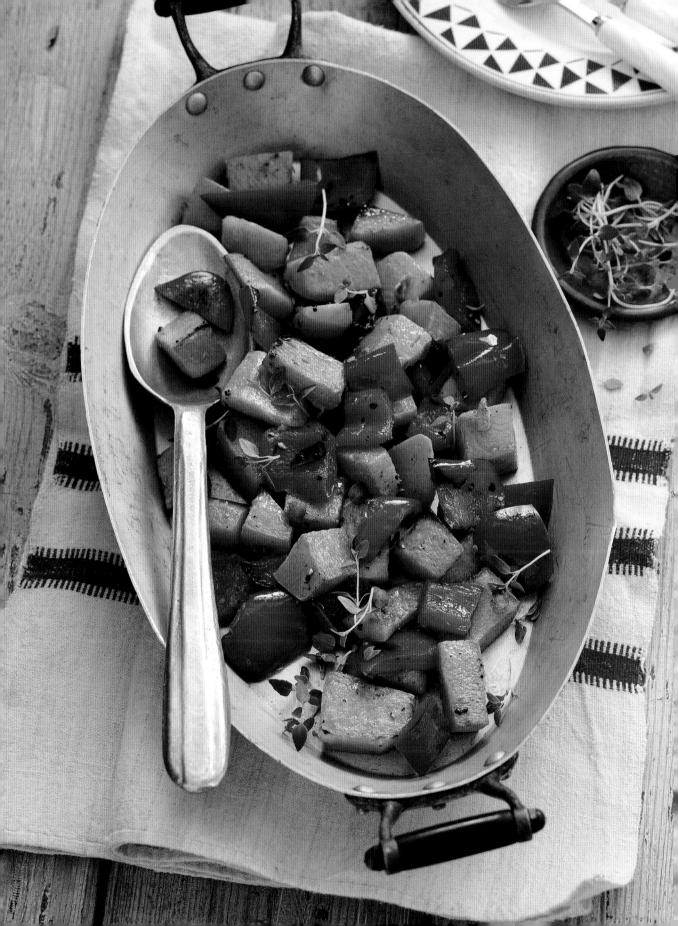

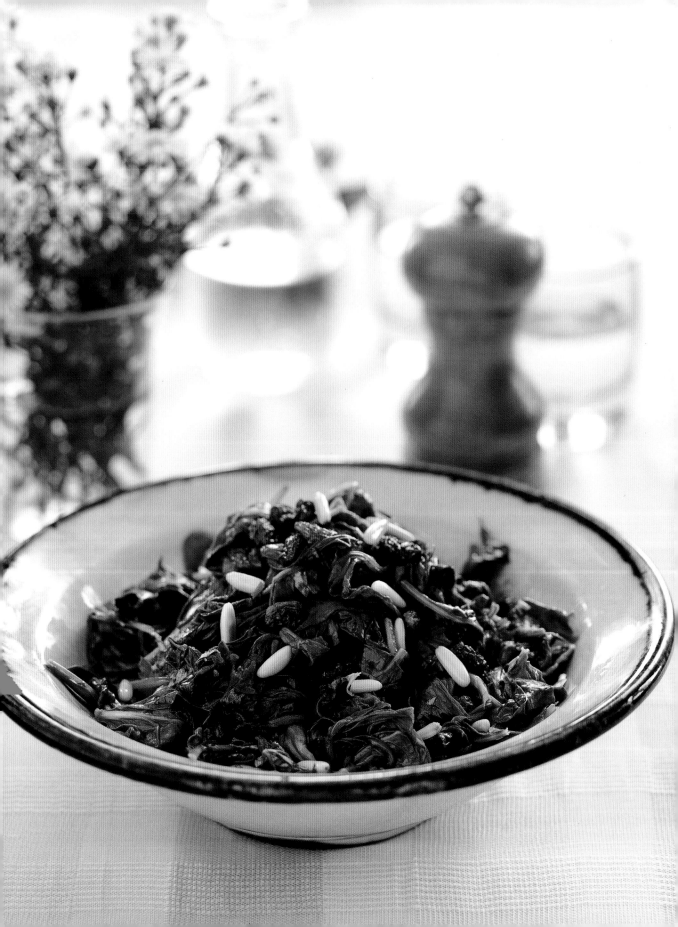

Sautéed spinach with raisins

SERVES 4

EASY Ⓥ ❄

Syns per serving
Extra Easy: ½ Syn
Original: ½ Syn
Green: ½ Syn

Preparation time: 10 minutes
plus soaking
Cooking time: less than 10 minutes

1 level tbsp raisins or golden sultanas
800g/1lb 12oz fresh spinach
low calorie cooking spray
3 tbsp finely chopped parsley
a pinch of grated nutmeg
salt and freshly ground black pepper
toasted pine nuts, to garnish (optional)

This Ligurian speciality of sautéed spinach makes a wonderful side dish, or you can toss it with cooked rice to turn it into a hearty lunch.

Soak the raisins or sultanas in a bowl of warm water for 20 minutes and then drain.

Meanwhile, wash the spinach leaves and drain well in a colander.

Spray a large non-stick frying pan with low calorie cooking spray and place over a medium heat. Add the spinach, parsley, nutmeg and drained raisins or sultanas and stir-fry for 6–8 minutes or until the spinach is wilted.

Season well and serve immediately garnished with toasted pine nuts (5 Syns per level tbsp), if desired.

Rosemary roasties

SERVES 4

EASY

Syns per serving
Extra Easy: Free
Green: Free
Original: 8 Syns

Preparation time: 15 minutes
Cooking time: under 40 minutes

6 medium potatoes (King Edwards
or Desiree), peeled and
cut into 2cm/¾in pieces
sea salt
low calorie cooking spray
1 garlic bulb, cloves separated
but unpeeled
2 tbsp fresh rosemary, finely chopped

Rosemary and garlic add a flavour-twist to these delicious Italian roast potatoes that will make a great accompaniment to any dish.

Preheat the oven to 200°C/Gas 6. Line a baking sheet with non-stick baking parchment.

Place the potatoes into a saucepan of boiling water with a couple of pinches of sea salt and simmer for about 10 minutes.

Remove the potatoes from the pan, drain well and pat dry with kitchen towel. Then place them in a single layer on the baking sheet. Spray with low calorie cooking spray and scatter over the garlic cloves and the rosemary.

Roast in the oven for 20–25 minutes or until golden. Remove from the oven, discard the garlic and serve immediately.

Stir-fried cabbage with fennel seeds and chilli

SERVES 4

EASY

Syns per serving
Extra Easy: Free
Original: Free
Green: Free

Preparation time: 15 minutes
Cooking time: under 20 minutes

1 large Savoy cabbage
low calorie cooking spray
2 garlic cloves, peeled and thinly sliced
2 tsp fennel seeds
1 tsp dried red chilli flakes
salt

This recipe uses the classic Italian technique for cooking leafy greens; first you blanch them and then stir-fry them with whatever seasonings you like. If you can get your hands on cavalo nero (very dark-leaf Italian cabbage), use it instead of the Savoy cabbage.

Trim the Savoy cabbage and separate the leaves, removing any tough stalks. Roughly chop the leaves.

Bring a large saucepan of lightly salted water to the boil. Add the cabbage leaves and cook for 6–7 minutes. Drain thoroughly in a colander.

Spray a large non-stick frying pan with low calorie cooking spray and place over a low heat. Add the garlic, fennel and chilli flakes and stir-fry for 2–3 minutes.

Stir in the cabbage, season with salt and stir-fry for 3–4 minutes or until wilted and well coated with the garlic mixture.

Serve immediately.

Courgette, Parmesan and mint cakes

SERVES 4

EASY ❄

Syns per serving
Extra Easy: 1½ Syns
Original: 1½ Syns
Green: 1½ Syns

Preparation time: 30 minutes
Cooking time: under 1 hour

low calorie cooking spray
6 spring onions, trimmed and
finely sliced
1 red chilli, deseeded and
finely chopped
500g/1lb 2oz courgettes,
coarsely grated
1 garlic clove, peeled and
finely chopped
salt and freshly ground black pepper
6 tbsp finely chopped mint
3 medium eggs
100g/3½oz fat free
natural fromage frais
4 level tbsp finely grated
Parmesan cheese

Delicious courgettes, grated and mixed with spring onions, chilli, mint and Parmesan cheese, make these delightful 'cakes' the perfect accompaniment to any chicken, meat or fish dish.

Spray a large frying pan with low calorie cooking spray and place over a medium heat. Add the spring onions and chilli and stir-fry for 1–2 minutes.

Squeeze out any excess liquid from the grated courgettes and add to the pan with the garlic. Cook for 15–20 minutes, stirring often, until the courgettes are completely wilted, making sure any liquid released is evaporated. Remove from the heat, season well and stir in the mint.

Preheat the oven to 180°C/Gas 4.

Lightly beat together the eggs with the fromage frais and the Parmesan cheese. Season well and stir into the courgette mixture. Divide the mixture into 8 portions and form each one into a round shape.

Place on a baking sheet lined with baking parchment and spray with low calorie cooking spray. Bake in the oven for 20–25 minutes or until firm.

Remove from the oven and allow to rest for 10 minutes before serving.

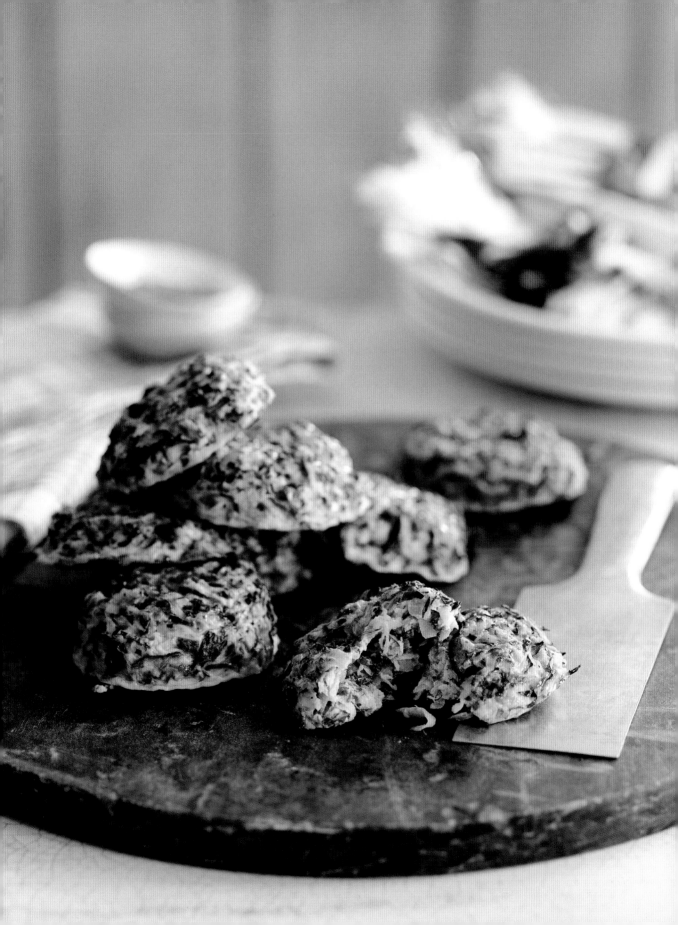

Braised borlotti beans

SERVES 4

EASY Ⓥ

Syns per serving
Extra Easy: Free
Green: Free
Original: 10½ Syns

Preparation time: 10 minutes plus
soaking
Cooking time: under 2 hours

250g/9oz dried borlotti beans
1 rosemary sprig
1 red chilli
2 bay leaves
1 onion, peeled and quartered
1 carrot, peeled and chopped
2 celery sticks, chopped
a small handful of wild rocket leaves
juice of 1 lemon
salt

Borlotti beans are widely eaten in Italy and they make a great addition to any table. You can substitute the borlotti beans with dried cannellini beans in this recipe.

Soak the beans in a large saucepan of cold water for 12–24 hours. Drain well and return to the pan.

Add the rosemary, red chilli, bay leaves, onion, carrot and celery. Pour over enough water to cover by 3cm/1¼in.

Bring to the boil and simmer for approximately 1½ hours or until the beans are soft. You will need to top up the water from time to time.

When the beans are cooked, remove the vegetables, herbs and red chilli. Chop up and deseed (optional) the red chilli and discard the rest.

Add the chopped chilli to the beans. Stir through the rocket and lemon juice and season well with salt before serving.

Fagioli all'uccelletto

SERVES 4

EASY

Syns per serving
Extra Easy: Free
Green: Free
Original: 8½ Syns

Preparation time: 10 minutes
Cooking time: under 15 minutes

low calorie cooking spray
2 garlic cloves, peeled and
finely chopped
1 red onion, peeled and finely chopped
4–5 sage leaves, chopped
2 x 400g cans cannellini beans,
drained and rinsed
4 tomatoes, skinned and chopped
salt and freshly ground black pepper

This wholesome and warming dish of cannellini beans with tomatoes and herbs is fresh and light, and is very good when served with grilled or baked chicken or fish.

Spray a large non-stick frying pan with low calorie cooking spray and place over a low heat. Add the garlic, onion and sage and stir-fry them for 6–8 minutes.

Add the cannellini beans and tomatoes and stir and cook for 4–5 minutes or until the beans have warmed through.

Season well and serve immediately.

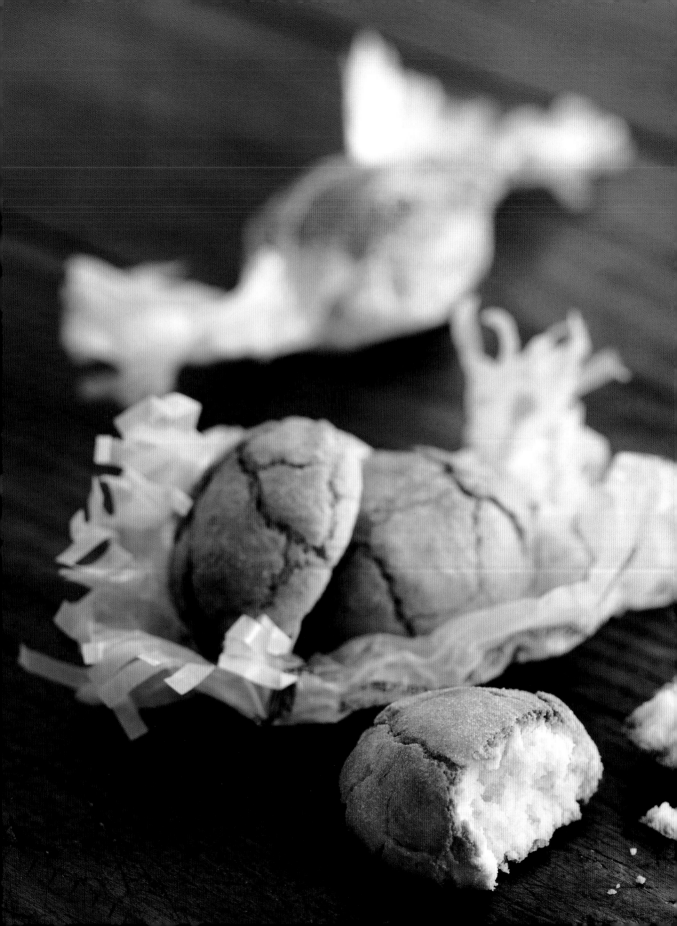

Chapter 8

Desserts

Gelato, semifreddo, sorbet, granita – with so many different words for iced desserts, it's no surprise that Italy is world famous for them! Made the Slimming World way, they can all still be on the menu when you're watching your weight. Everyone will love Instant Raspberry Sorbet and Strawberry Gelato (see pages 209 and 212), while Campari and Blood Orange Granita or Coffee Semifreddo are smart enough for entertaining (see pages 210 and 213). And we've also included some creamy Italian classics with a fruity twist – Peach Zabaglione, Raspberry Pannacotta and Chocolate Banana Tiramisu are recipes you'll turn to again and again (see pages 216, 219 and 220).

Strawberries with balsamic vinegar

750g/1lb 10oz ripe strawberries
2 tbsp artificial sweetener
2 tbsp aged balsamic vinegar
100g/3½oz fat free natural fromage
frais, to serve (optional)

Though at first it might seem an odd combination, the tart, rich balsamic vinegar really enhances the flavour of the strawberries. This is a perfect dessert for al fresco entertaining.

Wipe the strawberries with a clean, damp cloth and hull them. Then cut the strawberries in half and place in a wide bowl and sprinkle over the sweetener. Toss to coat evenly, cover and leave to macerate for 20–30 minutes.

Spoon the strawberries into individual dessert glasses and drizzle over the balsamic vinegar. Top with the fromage frais, if using, and serve immediately.

Figs baked with vanilla and amaretti

SERVES 4

EASY Ⓥ

Syns per serving
Extra Easy: 4½ Syns
Original: 4½ Syns
Green: 4½ Syns

Preparation time: 10 minutes
Cooking time: 10 minutes

12 large, ripe figs
2 soft, plump vanilla pods
4 amaretti biscuits
1 tbsp artificial sweetener
finely grated zest and juice of 1 lemon
fat free natural fromage frais, to serve

Delicious ripe figs are eaten all over Italy and here they are filled with a vanilla, lemon and amaretti biscuit mixture before being quickly baked. Take care not to overcook them or they will collapse.

Preheat the oven to 220°C/Gas 7.

Cut a deep cross in the top of each fig, so that they open up a little, and set aside.

Chop the vanilla pods and place in a small food processor with the amaretti biscuits, sweetener and lemon zest and pulse until roughly mixed.

Place the figs, cut sides up, in an ovenproof dish to fit snugly.

Using a small spoon, stuff the vanilla mixture into the figs and scatter over any remaining mixture. Squeeze over the lemon juice and place in the oven for 10 minutes.

Remove from the oven and allow to cool for a few minutes before serving with a dollop of the fromage frais.

Pears with honey and Pecorino

SERVES 4

REALLY EASY

Syns per serving
Extra Easy: 8 Syns
Original: 8 Syns
Green: 8 Syns

Preparation time: 10 minutes
Cooking time: none

4 ripe pears
110g/4oz Pecorino cheese
4 level tbsp runny honey
chopped walnuts, to serve (optional)

A typical Italian custom is to round off a meal with a combination of cheese, fruit and honey. The contrast of saltiness and sweetness is wonderful. You could substitute the Pecorino for a creamy Italian Dolcelatte cheese, if you prefer.

Peel, quarter and core the pears, then cut into thin wedges and arrange on individual plates.

Shave the Pecorino cheese using a vegetable peeler and also divide between the plates.

Drizzle over the honey and scatter over chopped walnuts (5 Syns per level tbsp), if using, and serve immediately.

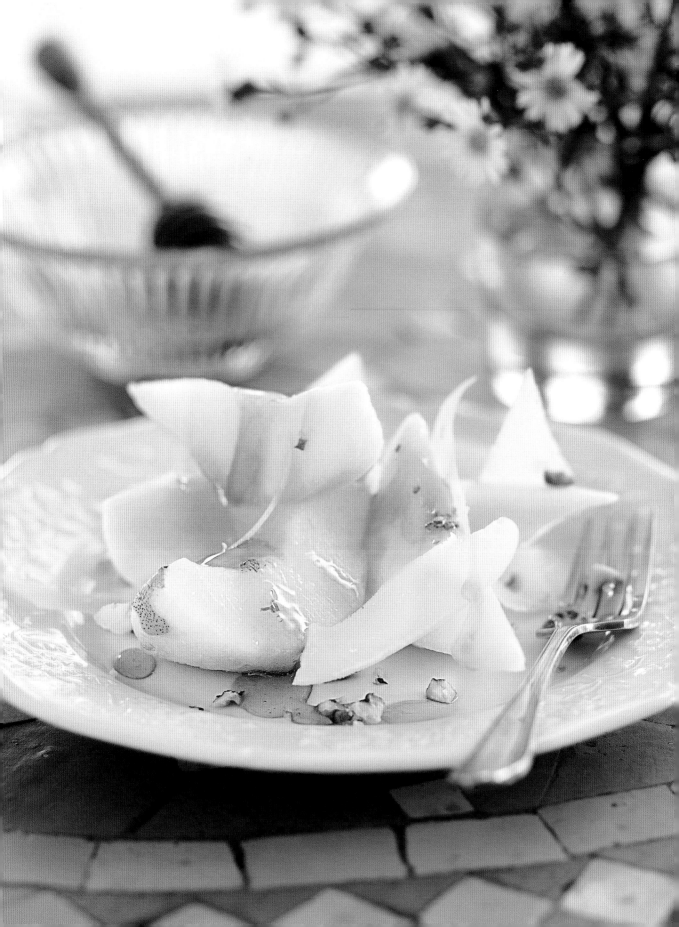

Watermelon and mandarin granita

SERVES 4

EASY Ⓥ

Syns per serving
Extra Easy: 4½ Syns
Original: 4½ Syns
Green: 4½ Syns

Preparation time: 20 minutes
plus freezing
Cooking time: none

600g/1lb 5oz watermelon flesh
4–5 tbsp artificial sweetener
finely grated zest of 1 mandarin
juice of 4 mandarins

Use the ripest, freshest fruit for this beautifully coloured ice treat, which is really refreshing on a hot summer's day.

Remove any seeds from the watermelon flesh and roughly chop it up.

Place in a blender or food processor with the sweetener, mandarin zest and juice and blend until fairly smooth.

Transfer the mixture to a shallow freezerproof container. Cover and freeze for 5–6 hours, beating the mixture with a fork every 30–40 minutes. Freeze until firm.

Remove from the freezer and place in the fridge for 15 minutes to soften. Using a fork, scrape the granita into chilled serving bowls or glasses and serve immediately.

Instant raspberry sorbet

SERVES 4

REALLY EASY ❆

Syns per serving
Extra Easy: 1½ Syns
Original: 1½ Syns
Green: 1½ Syns

Preparation time: 10 minutes
Cooking time: none

400g pack frozen raspberries
2 x 190g pots Müllerlight Vanilla Yogurt
(or fat free vanilla yogurt)
3 tbsp artificial sweetener
fresh raspberries, to garnish

This wonderfully quick, zingy sorbet can be made right before serving as it takes just minutes.

Place the frozen berries in a food processor with the yogurt and sweetener.

Whizz until well blended, making sure the fruit still has some texture. Scrape the mixture from the sides and blend again.

Spoon into chilled glasses or bowls and serve immediately, garnished with fresh raspberries.

Campari and blood orange granita

SERVES 4

EASY Ⓥ ❄

Syns per serving
Extra Easy: 4½ Syns
Original: 4½ Syns
Green: 4½ Syns

Preparation time: 20 minutes
plus freezing
Cooking time: none

500ml/18fl oz blood orange juice
2 tbsp Campari
4 tbsp artificial sweetener
2 large oranges, segmented
mint leaves, to garnish (optional)

Italian blood orange juice is widely available in most supermarkets. If you can't find it, you can use regular orange juice instead. For a child-friendly version of this refreshing dessert, simply leave out the Campari.

Place the orange juice, Campari and sweetener in a medium-sized bowl and whisk until they are well combined.

Transfer this mixture to a freezerproof container measuring about 20 x 20 x 5cm/8 x 8 x 2in. Place the granita in the freezer for at least 6 hours until set (or overnight if time permits).

Place four dessert glasses in the freezer to chill.

To serve, divide the orange segments between the bases of the glasses. Using a fork, scrape the surface of the granita to form crystals.

Divide the granita among the dessert glasses and garnish with mint, if desired. Serve immediately.

Tip Try serving the granita piled into hollowed-out orange shells.

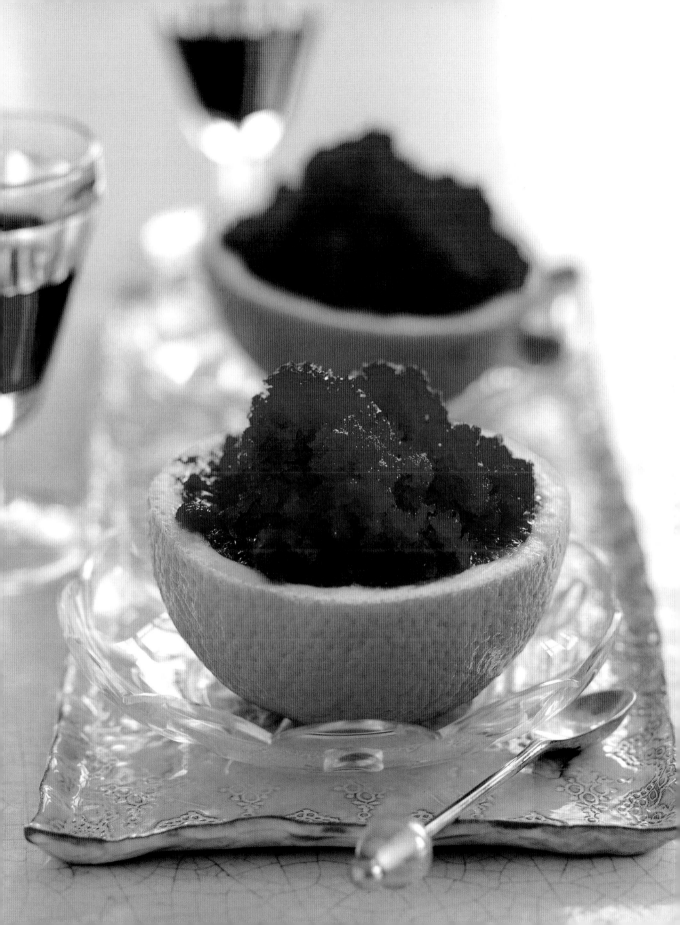

Strawberry gelato

SERVES 4

EASY

Syns per serving
Extra Easy: 4 Syns
Original: 4 Syns
Green: 4 Syns

Preparation time: 30 minutes plus
freezing
Cooking time: none

500g/1lb 2oz strawberries, plus extra to
garnish
3 tbsp artificial sweetener
2 large egg whites
200g/7oz low fat custard

All Italians love 'gelato' or ice cream and here we have a strawberry version that's really low in Syns compared to shop-bought varieties.

Wash, hull and roughly chop the strawberries. Place them in a food processor or liquidiser with the sweetener and blend until smooth.

Add the egg whites and custard and blend to combine.

Pour the mixture in to a shallow freezerproof container and freeze for 1 hour. Remove from the freezer and mash or whisk to break down any large crystals. Return the container to the freezer and freeze for at least 3 hours until solid.

Remove from freezer 10–20 minutes before serving. Scoop into chilled bowls or dessert glasses and garnish with fresh strawberries.

Tip You can use an ice-cream machine, if preferred for step 3; just follow the manufacturer's instructions.

Coffee semifreddo

WORTH THE EFFORT Ⓥ

Syns per serving
Extra Easy: 3½ Syns
Original: 3½ Syns
Green: 3½ Syns

Preparation time: 25 minutes
plus freezing
Cooking time: none

350g/12oz low fat custard
150g/5oz fat free natural fromage frais
1 tsp vanilla extract
4–5 tbsp artificial sweetener
3 large egg whites

FOR THE COFFEE SAUCE
200ml/7fl oz cold espresso coffee
2–3 tbsp artificial sweetener
2 tbsp coffee-flavoured liqueur,
e.g. Tia Maria (optional)

Typical of the Italian region of Emilia-Romagna, semifreddo literally means 'half-cold'. Here we have a wonderful custard and coffee-flavoured pud.

Place the custard and fromage frais in a large mixing bowl. Add the vanilla extract and sweetener and stir to mix well.

In a separate bowl whisk the egg whites until stiff and then gently fold them into the custard mixture using a metal spoon.

Line a medium-sized loaf tin with cling film. Spoon the mixture into the tin, cover with cling film and place in the freezer for 6–8 hours until firm (or overnight if time permits).

Meanwhile heat the coffee in a small saucepan, add the sweetener and stir until dissolved. Add the coffee-flavoured liqueur (2 Syns per tbsp), if using, and boil vigorously or until syrupy. Remove from the heat and set aside.

About 20 minutes before serving, transfer the semifreddo from the freezer to the fridge.

Turn out onto a serving plate and cut into thick slices. Spoon over the coffee sauce, which can be warm or at room temperature.

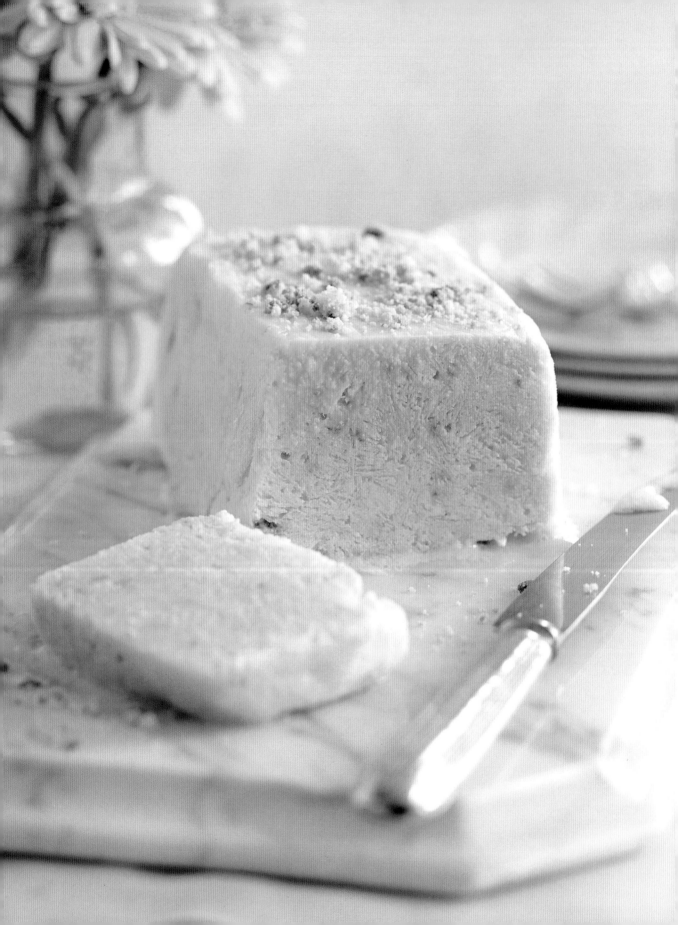

Almond and amaretti terrine

SERVES 4

WORTH THE EFFORT (V) (❄)

Syns per serving
Extra Easy: 7 Syns
Original: 7 Syns
Green: 7 Syns

Preparation time: 25 minutes plus freezing
Cooking time: none

400g/14oz low fat custard
100g/3½oz fat free natural fromage frais
2 tsp almond essence
4–5 tbsp artificial sweetener
3 large egg whites
8 amaretti biscuits

Amaretti are little Italian biscuits made with ground almonds. They add a wonderful texture and flavour to this delicious frozen dessert.

Place the custard and fromage frais in a large mixing bowl. Add the almond essence and sweetener and stir to mix well.

In a separate bowl whisk the egg whites until stiff, then gently fold them into the custard mixture using a metal spoon.

Roughly crush 7 of the amaretti biscuits and stir into the custard mixture.

Line a medium-sized loaf tin with cling film. Spoon the mixture into the tin, cover with cling film and freeze for 6–8 hours until firm (or overnight if time permits).

About 20 minutes before serving transfer the terrine from the freezer to the fridge. Turn the terrine out onto a serving plate, crumble over the remaining biscuit, cut into thick slices and serve immediately.

Peach zabaglione

SERVES 4

WORTH THE EFFORT Ⓥ

Syns per serving
Extra Easy: ½ Syn
Original: ½ Syn
Green: ½ Syn

Preparation time: 10 minutes
Cooking time: 8–10 minutes

4 ripe peaches
4 large egg yolks
2 tbsp sweet Marsala wine
4 tbsp artificial sweetener
savoiardi or sponge fingers,
to serve (optional)

There is nothing quite as deliciously sensual as warm zabaglione served straight from the pan. The secret is not to let the mixture get too hot, but still warm enough to cook and thicken the yolk into a creamy mixture. Make this at the last moment, just before serving, as it doesn't take long and is well worth the effort.

Peel, halve and stone the peaches and cut into thick slices. Divide the slices between four dessert glasses, reserving a few for decoration.

Place the egg yolks, Marsala wine and sweetener in a medium-sized heatproof bowl and beat with an electric whisk until well blended.

Place the bowl over a saucepan of gently simmering water, making sure the bottom does not touch the water or the eggs will scramble.

Whisk for 8–10 minutes or until the mixture is glossy, pale, light and fluffy and holds a trail.

Spoon immediately over the peach slices and serve with the reserved peach slices and sponge fingers (1 Syn each), if using.

Tip To make a chilled version, remove the bowl from the heat and keep whisking until the mixture is completely cool. Spoon into the glasses and chill for 3–4 hours before serving.

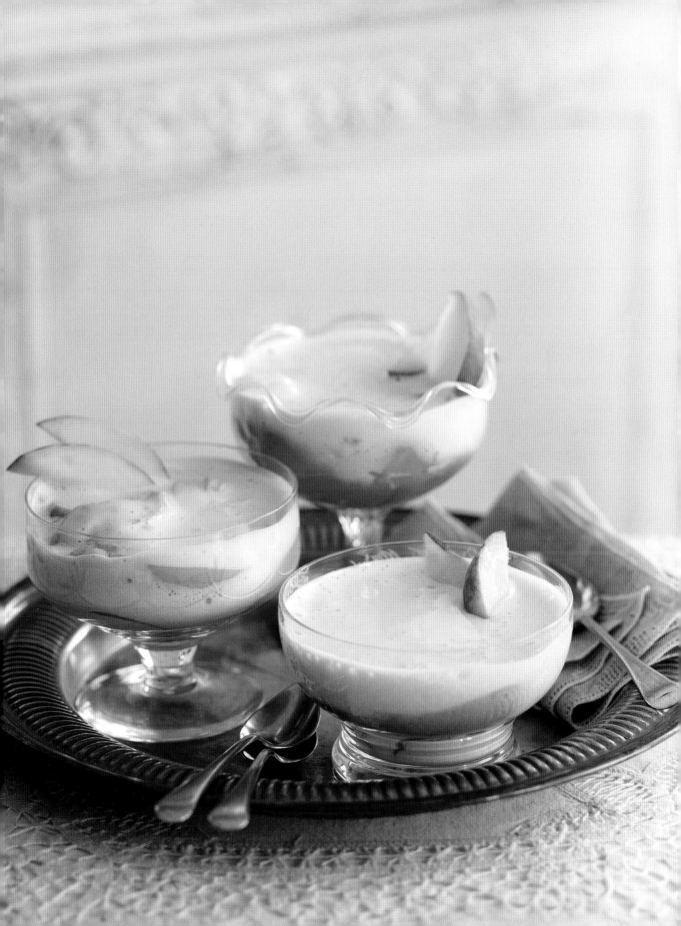

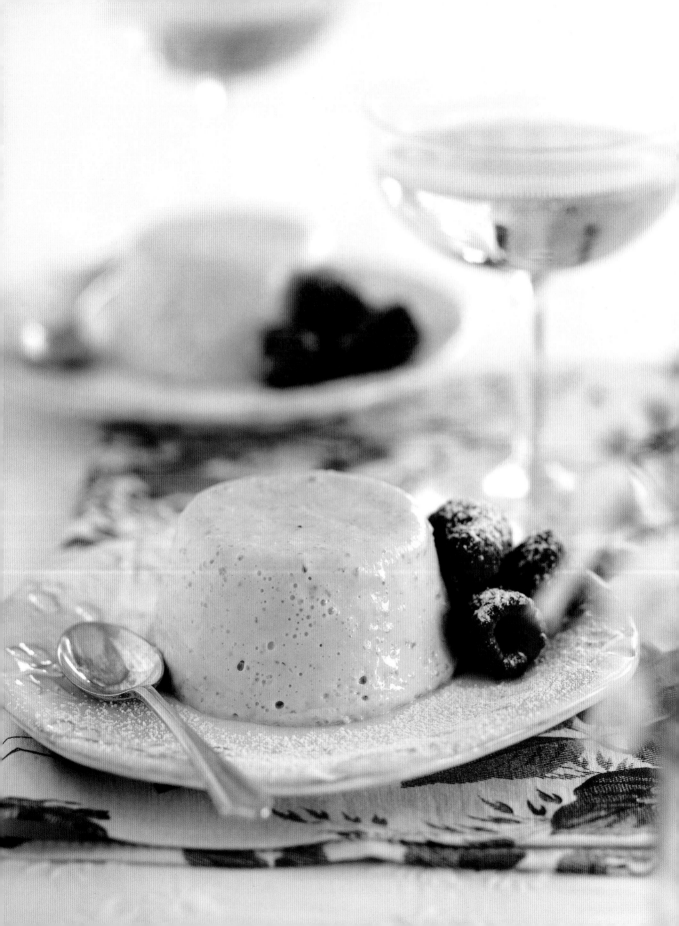

Raspberry pannacotta

SERVES 4

EASY

Syns per serving
Extra Easy: ½ Syn
Original: ½ Syn
Green: ½ Syn

Preparation time: 20 minutes
plus chilling
Cooking time: none

100g/3½oz fresh raspberries,
plus extra to garnish
100g/3½oz quark
5 tbsp artificial sweetener
1 tsp vanilla extract
2 x 190g pots Müllerlight Raspberry
and Cranberry Yogurt
1 x 15g sachet gelatine
1 large egg white
mint leaves, to garnish (optional)

Usually made with double cream,
this delicious Italian dessert is given
a low-Syn twist by using quark and fat
free fruit yogurt instead.

Place the raspberries in a large fine metal sieve over a bowl and press down with the back of a spoon to extract the pulp and juices. Discard the remaining seeds.

Place the quark, sweetener, vanilla extract and yogurt into a food processor and stir in the raspberry mixture.

Place 8 tablespoons of hot water in a small heatproof bowl and sprinkle over the gelatine. Stand the bowl in a saucepan of hot water and stir until the gelatine has dissolved.

Add the gelatine to the quark and raspberry mixture and blend in the processor until smooth. Transfer to a bowl.

Beat the egg white until softly peaked and gently fold through the raspberry mixture using a metal spoon. Divide between individual moulds and chill in the fridge for 6–8 hours until set (or overnight if time permits).

Dip the moulds in hot water for a few seconds to loosen the pannacotta and turn out onto serving plates. Serve garnished with reserved raspberries and mint leaves, if desired.

Chocolate banana tiramisu

SERVES 4–6

EASY Ⓥ ❄

Syns per serving (serves 4)
Extra Easy: 3½ Syns
Original: 3½ Syns
Green: 3½ Syns

Syns per serving (serves 6)
Extra Easy: 2 Syns
Original: 2 Syns
Green: 2 Syns

Preparation time: 25–30 minutes
plus chilling
Cooking time: none

200g/7oz quark
200g/7oz fat free natural fromage frais
1 tsp vanilla extract
3 tbsp artificial sweetener
150ml/5fl oz strong coffee, cooled
12 sponge fingers
4 ripe bananas, peeled and sliced
2 tsp cocoa powder
melted dark chocolate, to drizzle
(optional)

This delicious 'pick-me-up' dessert is an Italian favourite. Here it is given a twist with the addition of sliced bananas.

Beat together the quark, fromage frais and vanilla extract in a bowl. Add the sweetener and stir well to mix.

Pour the cooled coffee into a shallow bowl. Dip the sponge fingers briefly into the coffee, layering half of them in the base of a medium-sized dessert bowl measuring about 20 x 15cm/8 x 6in, or individual serving glasses.

Top with half of the fromage frais mixture, then lay the banana slices on top of the fromage frais.

Add another layer of sponge fingers and top with the remaining fromage frais mixture.

Cover and chill in the fridge for 3–4 hours until ready to serve.

Just before serving, dust with the cocoa powder and drizzle with the melted chocolate (4 Syns per level tbsp), if using.

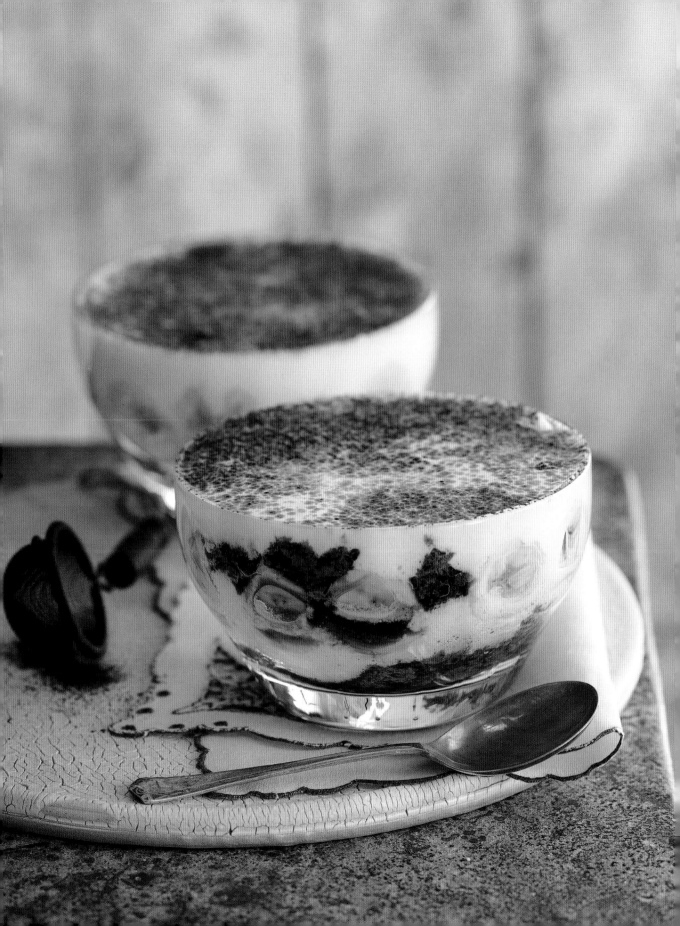

Index